"Innovative, informative and transformative, Durrani's research and creation of the model, S-BRATA, is a must read for art therapists working with people on the autism spectrum."

Emily Nolan, DAT, ATR-BC, LPC, assistant professor at Mount Mary University

"Dr. Huma Durrani makes a significant contribution to the knowledge base of Autism Spectrum Disorder with this book. She is a mother, a scientist, and a clinician and has masterfully combined her observational skills and wisdom to develop the S-BRATA. Durrani offers a compassionate presentation of her struggles and trials with her own son, who has ASD, that led to this process. She supports the S-BRATA with strong theory from scientific method, developmental theory, and art therapy. Durrani's S-BRATA brings a valuable treatment and intervention to clinicians working with people with ASD. Brava!"

Beth Gonzalez-Dolginko, EdD, LCAT, ATR-BC, author of *Art Therapy with Adults with Autism Spectrum Disorder*

"As a skilled clinician, art therapist, and mother of a grown child on the autism spectrum, Dr. Durrani contributes a critical 'missing piece' that will make therapy much more effective: an emotionally attuned relationship that is communicated in the language of the senses. With the S-BRATA model, she demonstrates how art therapists not only introduce a world of creative materials to children with sensory challenges but use them to build a reciprocal, social relationship on the child's terms. This excellent text contributes considerably to autism treatment with clinician-led research written with the empathic knowledge of a parent. As such, it is important reading for clinicians and parents alike, attuning both to the needs of the child—beyond behavioural fixes and toward a real capacity for social and emotional connection."

Lynn Kapitan, PhD, HLM, ATR-BC, professor at Mount Mary University, past-president of AATA, and author of *Introduction to Art Therapy Research (2nd ed.).*

Sensory-Based Relational Art Therapy Approach (S-BRATA)

This book bridges art therapy practice and research by presenting Sensory-Based Relational Art Therapy Approach (S-BRATA), a clinically tested framework for working with children with autism spectrum disorder (ASD) that explicitly addresses sensory dysfunction and its impact on impaired attachment.

The author shows how art therapy can facilitate attachment while addressing sensory problems that might underlie impaired attachment, shifting the focus from the behavioral to the emotional development of the child with autism. The book additionally challenges traditional aspects of art therapy practice, particularly the focus on the relational aspect of the intervention and not the art product. Not restrictive or prescriptive and with the potential to be adapted to other interventions, S-BRATA provides an explicit framework for doing art therapy with children on the spectrum that opens the scope of art therapy practice and encourages flexibility and adaptation.

Clinicians, students and parents alike will benefit from the text's clear outline for relational development with individuals on the spectrum and its emphasis on the importance of the psycho-emotional health of a child with ASD.

Huma Durrani, DAT, is an art therapist and practice-based researcher who owns Coloured Canvas, a specialized community resource for individual and group art therapy for children and adolescents with autism spectrum disorder, psycho-emotional and behavioural issues in Singapore.

Sensory-Based Relational Art Therapy Approach (S-BRATA)

Supporting Psycho-Emotional Needs in Children with Autism

Huma Durrani

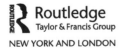
Routledge
Taylor & Francis Group

NEW YORK AND LONDON

First published 2021
by Routledge
52 Vanderbilt Avenue, New York, NY 10017

and by Routledge
2 Park Square, Milton Park, Abingdon, Oxon, OX14 4RN

Routledge is an imprint of the Taylor & Francis Group, an informa business

Library of Congress Cataloging-in-Publication Data
Names: Durrani, Huma, author.
Title: Sensory-based relational art therapy approach (S-BRATA) :
supporting psycho-emotional needs in children with autism/Huma
Durrani.
Description: New York, NY : Routledge, 2021. | Includes
bibliographical references and index. | Identifiers: LCCN 2020033307
(print) | LCCN 2020033308 (ebook) | ISBN 9780367442279 (hbk)
| ISBN 9780367442262 (pbk) | ISBN 9781003008422 (ebk)
Subjects: LCSH: Art therapy. | Children with autism spectrum
disorders.
Classification: LCC RC489.A7 D87 2021 (print) | LCC RC489.A7
(ebook) | DDC 616.89/1656--dc23
LC record available at https://lccn.loc.gov/2020033307
LC ebook record available at https://lccn.loc.gov/2020033308

ISBN: 978-0-367-44227-9 (hbk)
ISBN: 978-0-367-44226-2 (pbk)
ISBN: 978-1-003-00842-2 (ebk)

Typeset in Goudy
by MPS Limited, Dehradun

Contents

List of Figures

Foreword

Chris Belkofer

In my first years as a new practitioner conducting group and individual art therapy with children and adolescents in residential care, I don't think I remained seated for longer than 15 minutes out of my eight-hour day. Prior to my training in art therapy, I worked in the service industry as a waiter for over ten years. At the end of the day, both professions left me with a sore back, tired feet and sometimes messy clothes. Upon entering art therapy graduate school, like many people, I imagined therapy happened in tidy offices. I imagined mental health therapy sessions consisted of people sitting on couches sandwiched between decorative throw pillows or maybe in an awkward circle of stiff-backed chairs. Therapists wore nice suits and paint-free sweaters. I really wish I had this book back then.

Even as my studies progressed in graduate school as I learned more about "non-traditional" art therapy spaces and studio based approaches (C. Moon, 2004), I still maintained a belief that art therapy and mental health were a primarily sedentary kind of work, low on kinesthetics and high on contemplation. Like many, I worked from a basic conceptual model that an art therapy session, like all mental health sessions, followed a basic order of operations: client enters session, client sits down at art table, client makes an image, therapist and client talk about image as related to client's life, therapist and client clean up the art therapy room and client leaves the session. To modify or defer from this structure was to be engaging in something potentially therapeutic but not "real" therapy. I really wish I had this book back then.

A few months on the job as a new professional quickly expanded my previous expectations of what therapy was supposed to look like, to feel like and to be like. The creativity as well as the unique needs of my clients required I had to expand my approach and to rethink my previous assumptions. Metaphorically speaking, I learned that many of the children and adolescents I served were not only disinterested in coloring within the lines, most were more inclined to throw out the entire piece of paper. Their innovation and creativity liberated me from my earlier notions of art making process and product and introduced me to a new kind of full body approach to art making. But I still struggled how to explain what I was doing to my psychodynamically oriented clinical supervisor. I really wish I had this book back then.

My work with this population was dynamic, to say the least, and never boring. The tone and the feel of the sessions would shift moment by moment with multiple scenes and acts to be witnessed. It was genuinely hard for me to keep up at times, which could be both scary and inspiring. There was so much to process in these documented 50 minutes. Time could pass like seconds or drag at a snail's pace. My clients taught (really demanded) me to be present. If I drifted off and attention waned, I could miss a season of change. Fall could turn to winter, winter could shift to summer and, somehow, I would end up in spring. I would live a calendar of weather patterns in just one session.

The art made with and among my clients encouraged me to recontextualize definitions of art media and freed me from art school training and traditions. This approach to art making also seemed to help me and my clients grow closer and develop a strong therapeutic rapport in a way that remains to this day still hard to articulate or explain. In addition to rethinking how I defined visual art, I also began to re-evaluate how I approached developing, creating and staging the therapeutic space. I had to let go of previous notions of control, expertise, proximity and stillness. It's funny how a seven-year-old can inspire you to completely rethink your approach to what works in therapy. Somewhat rudimentary questions such as where to sit, how long to sit, what media to use and what art directives if any were needed (all that stuff I had to just throw out the window) buttressed up against more layered reflections regarding foundational assumptions of the work.

How does experiential learning and shared experiences form interpersonal relationships? Where does effective therapy happen? How do we flow together? How do I translate the value of this work to other professionals? How can I make the damn tape and foil sculpture of Sponge Bob Square Pants stand up straight?!? What is the nature of human attachment? It's funny how a seven-year-old can inspire you to existential doubt. In short, a few months into my career and I basically had to reimagine everything I was taught. That was over 15 years ago. Needless to say, I really wish I had this book then.

Art therapy is continually in the process of definition, conceptualization and reinvention. Even as the field rapidly progresses, foundational questions remain. It is widely understood that art therapy provides a model for working with clients whom traditional talk therapy may not benefit (Moon & Belkofer, 2014). But Durrani pushes this even further, providing a framework to effectively work with persons for whom traditional art therapy approaches might not work either. In this pioneering text, the author illustrates numerous theories related to art therapy, including but not limited to nonverbal process-oriented therapeutic attunement, the role of sensory and kinaesthetic processes in art therapy and approaches to treatment with clients on the autism spectrum.

The enthusiasm for how to apply brain and body-based approaches to art therapy treatment continues to grow, but there still remains a need for guidance and applications of these potentials. This text builds off the growing literature in art therapy that has employed neuroscience frameworks as a foundational underpinning of practice (Chapman, 2014; Hass-Cohen, 2008; Hass-Cohen & Findlay, 2015; King, 2016; Lusebrink, 2004). Building upon this base, Huma Durrani specializes in taking a deeper look at how neuroscience and attachment theory can be utilized in art therapy work with neurodivergent populations. In this book, she specializes on working with clients on the autism spectrum, an underserved and under-researched group. At the core of the work is an exploration of neurodiversity that illustrates how therapeutic art making can address the sensory deficit disorders associated with individuals on the spectrum to improve attachment patterns.

The book begins with a detailed exploration of autism spectrum disorder (ASD), childhood attachment and neurodevelopmental theory and how sensory integration disorder (SID) impacts the relational dyad between caregiver and child. Rather than viewing persons who may present with ASD features as incapable of forming healthy attachments, this integrated model expands upon traditionally narrow views of both working and conceptualizing persons with neurodiverse backgrounds. Durrani lays out a convincing argument, based on her own experiences as a mother of a neurodiverse child, that current models of autism treatment overemphasize behavioral modification at the expense of the child's emotional well-being and relational development. She articulates how the struggles that may present related to attachment are not related to a lack of a desire or need to attune and interpersonally connect but rather are related to the sensory disruptions that can make such connections physically painful. The author eloquently outlines her own experiences as a parent and how these dynamics contributed to her own feelings of mis-attunement between her and her son. She identifies the circle of disconnect associated with SID as a barrier in establishing healthy attachment relationships between caregiver and child. The caregiver feels unsuccessful as the child struggles to manage their internal experiences of closeness inherent in the bond. Without a working understanding of the unique sensational world of the child, the caregiver may be set up as they naturally interpret the infant's dysregulation as a personal failure.

In the next chapter, Durrani provides strong rationale for how process-oriented approaches to art therapy that address underlying sensory dysregulation can at the same time help to improve interpersonal connections. She outlines how by attending to the sensory needs of the clients, the therapist is attending to their emotional needs as well. Such attention is essential to develop a relational bond/attachment. In this chapter, the reader is fully introduced to Durrani's Sensory-Based Relational Art Therapy Approach (S-BRATA), which utilizes nonverbal and sensory dependent art making processes to promote interactions and build attachment. Durrani illustrates how by attuning to the individual differences related to thresholds of sensory stimulation, the therapist can tailor an individualized approach to treatment. This approach is a welcomed addition to existing art therapy literature by Chapman (2014), Hass-Cohen (2008) and others (Hass-Cohen & Carr, 2008;

King, 2016; Malchiodi, 2006, 2020) that identifies the brain as central to relationally informed–based approaches to art therapy. Durrani expands upon the growing work within art therapy that has integrated neuroscience theory into practice by exploring an approach that, while not limited to, is uniquely applicable to the ASD population.

The remaining chapters illustrate a grounded theory methodology that informed the creation of the S-BRATA and provide rich case vignettes to illustrate how this model is applied in practice, culminating with seven themes of S-BRATA and recommendations for future research and development. While beneficial to anyone working with neurodiverse populations, these chapters elucidate a relational model for how to facilitate a therapeutic relationship through sensory and experiential experience. The author builds off her personal and professional experience as well as the recent developments in art therapy that emphasize neuroscience as a way to conceptualize art therapy and promote what Hass-Cohen and Findlay (2015) described as "participatory meaning-making experiences" (p. 2).

In summary, this book is an essential read for those who work with challenging populations and who have sought a model and clinical rationale for how to work with clients who are nonverbal and in a "traditional way." The information contained herein will help art therapists remain grounded even when working with patients that challenge the notion. No doubt many other professionals will benefit from this book as well. Practitioners who are looking for models of how to apply sensory-based and process-based work in a clinical setting will find much to apply here. In addition, the emphasis on considering the role of the body and sensory processing as a means for relationship building when working with neuro-atypical clients is a significant contribution to approaches to autism research and autism treatment in general. One need not be an art therapist to gain a greater sense for how art making can be used with this population. Of particular impact is the author's connection of sensory processing related to early childhood attachment theory and the caregiver-child dyad. Her assertion that art therapy can address attachment patterns through sensory-based art making is significant step forward for art therapy and attachment theory in general.

Having worked personally with Huma as her doctoral instructor and advisor, I have been firsthand witness to her passion and clinical expertise. Our many conversations like the writings in this book have inspired me to think about ASD, neurodiversity, art therapy and interpersonal connections in a new way. I'm better for it, and I'm honored to share a little of this experience with you. I also must confess that our many talks together and the authentic vulnerability in allowing others such firsthand access to her clinical work have been validating to my previously mentioned new kid on the job as well as the expert professional who writes this today. Too often, case studies and clinical writings sparkle a bit too brightly with a sheen of certainty. By contrast, Huma does not refrain from sharing with us what was not working as well. It is rare for clinicians to so fully let us into their process. In this book, she documents not just her successes but also the times she was met with indifference, reluctance and fear and the many periods of limited to no progress. I'm excited for you to experience her story and her vision. I am really glad we have this book.

References

Chapman, L. (2014). *Neurobiologically informed trauma therapy with children and adolescents: Understanding mechanisms of change.* New York, NY: W. W. Norton & Company.

Hass-Cohen, N. (2008). Partnering of art therapy and neuroscience. In Hass-Cohen, N. & Carr, R. (Eds.), *Art therapy and clinical neuroscience* (pp. 21–42). London, England: Jessica Kingsley.

Hass-Cohen, N., & Carr, R. (Eds.). (2008). *Art therapy and clinical neuroscience.* London, England: Jessica Kingsley.

Hass-Cohen, N., & Findlay, C. J. (2015). *Art therapy and the neuroscience of relationships: Creativity and resiliency.* New York, NY: W. W. Norton & Company, Inc.

King, J. (Ed.) (2016). *Art therapy, trauma, and neuroscience: Theoretical and practical perspectives.* New York, NY: Routledge.

Lusebrink, V. B. (2004). Art therapy and the brain: An attempt to understand the underlying processes of art expression in therapy. *Art Therapy: Journal of the American Art Therapy Association, 21*(3), 125–135.

Malchiodi, C. A. (2006). Expressive therapies: History, theory, and practice. In Malchiodi, C. A. (Ed.), *Expressive therapies* (pp. 1–15). New York, NY: Guilford Press.

Malchiodi, C. A. (2020). *Trauma and expressive arts therapy: Brain, body, and imagination in the healing process.* New York, NY: Guildford Press.

Moon, B. L., & Belkofer, C. (2014). *Artist, therapist, and teacher: Selected writings by Bruce L. Moon.* Springfield, IL: Charles. C. Thomas.

Moon, C. H. (2002). *Studio art therapy: Cultivating the artist identity in the art therapist.* London: Jessica Kingsley

About the Author

Huma Durrani is a Pakistani Singaporean based in Singapore. She has professional and personal experience of almost two decades working with children and adolescents with differences, first as an educational therapist and then as an art therapist. Huma has conducted doctoral research on ASD and comorbid SID and has designed a framework for doing art therapy with children with autism, namely: Sensory-Based Relational Art Therapy Approach (S-BRATA). Huma has published her research in academic journals and presented her work internationally. She also published a memoir called "Wrapped in Blue" in which she documented her journey about raising her 22-year-old son with autism. Huma blogs regularly about art therapy, parenting and mental health.

Introduction

Moeez, my two-and-a-half-year-old son, lay on the cold marble floor pressing his knees and elbows deep into the hardness of the stone, lightly banging his forehead in synchrony with the persistent movement of his limbs. His *lying down* ritual, as I called it, coincided with the birth of my second child; hence, I assumed it was an expression of sibling rivalry. Moeez was not able to communicate verbally for lack of expressive language, and I watched him in vain, agonising over what appeared to be a painful ordeal, helpless at not being able to address the behavior. This *lying down* behavior could last for hours until Moeez was physically picked up and engaged otherwise. With a newborn child, it required an enormous amount of effort on my part to redirect Moeez's puzzling act and I vacillated between frustration and anxiety over his incomprehensible reaction and my misplaced presumption of its source. Moeez had till then not been diagnosed with autism, and since he was my first born, I was not awakened to the realisation of him being any different from other children until he was almost 3 years of age. By then, the absence of speech and lack reciprocal behaviors alerted me to the possibility of an underlying problem.

Finally, after Moeez was diagnosed with autism spectrum disorder (ASD), I was referred to an occupational therapist who was the first professional I saw in the context of Moeez's therapeutic needs. I had just moved to Singapore from Pakistan where autism was almost unheard of, and the former, too, was only just waking up to the pervasiveness of the disorder, and hence the lack of awareness coupled with insufficient resources in terms of intervention and support. Moeez's OT introduced me to sensory integration dysfunction (SID) and I learned a new terminology for the senses of smell: olfactory; touch: tactile; auditory: hearing; vestibular: movement and balance, and proprioception: sense of position and movement of the body, along with the familiar vocabulary for the senses of sight: visual and taste. Moeez's *lying down* behavior finally began to make sense even though initially I struggled with grasping the complexity of sensory regulation issues. His OT explained that the *lying down* ritual was instigated by an impairment in Moeez's proprioceptive system. Consequently, pushing his body into the floor enabled Moeez to obtain the input he required to feel his body parts. I found it hard to imagine how something like that was even possible ... to not know where your arm was or perhaps your nose or if you were sitting or floating. It dawned on me that Moeez was living a very different reality than I could perceive with my well-integrated sensory modalities I took for granted! Contrary to my uninformed hypothesis, Moeez's *lying down* was not an expression of anxiety; rather, it was his way of addressing that anxiety that emanated from a sensory system that was unable to coherently organize input from the environment. What I thought was pain inducing behavior was known as self-stimulatory behavior or *stimming* (*stim:* singular) in ASD vernacular. Children with autism stimmed or indulged in stereotypical behaviors that were repetitive and recurrent in order to instigate a pleasurable response from their nervous system. Through these stimming behaviors that may manifest as hand-flapping, spinning, rocking, jumping and so on, children with autism try to cope with overwhelming anxiety. As I became familiar with autism, the complexity of its etiology and the comorbidity of the challenges inherent in the spectrum, I began to see Moeez from a different perspective. It felt as if I was getting to know him all over again.

Dealing with Moeez's sensory issues and *stimming* remained one of the biggest challenges for our family for many years since some of his behaviors were socially inappropriate and potentially dangerous for him. Especially when he achieved puberty, the lying down *stim* could be misperceived as sexualised behavior as it resulted in undesirable consequences. A combination of occupational therapy (OT) and behavioral interventions helped Moeez manage his anxiety and channelize inappropriate *stimming* into more acceptable forms.

Moeez started talking at 6 years of age and well into his teens when he was able to express himself, he communicated why stimming was so important to him and how it helped him calm down. Moeez's stimming has reduced considerably over the years; however, it is very much a part of who he is.

My career path as a therapist developed hand in hand with my role as a caregiver. I had a degree in textile design from an art college in Pakistan but did not pursue it as a career since Moeez was born soon after I graduated. Following his diagnosis, I was immersed in caregiving for two children and a gruelling routine of therapies for Moeez. Finally, when I had some space to breathe, I chose to become an educational therapist as it seemed a natural progression from caregiving for a child with differences to working with similar children. I felt I had developed an innate capacity to connect with children who had different abilities and their caregivers. Thus, I taught literacy for many years to children with learning differences. It was during that period that I saw how creative expression came easily to children who otherwise struggled with reading and writing. I recall asking some of my students to draw and sing to learn spellings and recall sight words. I yearned to make art with them as I taught them phonology, wanting to connect with them at a deeper level. The Master's degree in art therapy from LASALLE College of Arts in Singapore came as the perfect opportunity for me to practice art as a form of therapy and turned out to be a life changing experience, not just professionally but personally as well. Interestingly, my very first research proposal at LASALLE focused on the regulatory aspect of art making. Perhaps I was intrinsically motivated to look for something that could address anxiety in children with autism, considering my history with Moeez. Little did I know that the seed for my future doctorate had been sowed in the first year of my Master's program.

After I graduated, ironically, I secured a job as an art therapist at an occupational therapy center where I provided art therapy to children with autism. Incidentally, I had wanted to work with trauma and abuse, but job opportunities for art therapists in Singapore were scarce in those days and one was lucky to find any work. My training in LASALLE had been heavily psychodynamic, and I was not sure how good a fit I would be in an OT environment, especially when I was explicitly asked to adapt to a more developmental approach. The shift from familiar ground, which meant exiting my comfort zone and switching perspective from implicit to explicit behaviors, was initially uncomfortable. Nevertheless, it was the best thing that could have happened since I was driven to focus on the sensory qualities of art materials and not so much the art product. Progressing from a decidedly psychodynamic stance to a developmental one allowed me to integrate my training with my life experience as the caregiver of a child with extreme sensory challenges. Sitting through countless hours of OT and behavioral interventions with Moeez had lent me considerable insight into sensory integration therapy, and I felt a sense of familiarity with the children at the OT center, most of who had severe sensory integration issues. Soon after starting work, I realised that in order to engage children with SID in any sort of art making or even to pay attention to me, I had to first address their level of anxiety. A lot of the anxiety seemed to stem from sensory challenges, something that I had learned from observing Moeez and later confirmed through research. I recalled how Moeez had been averse to communication or learning until his sensory needs had been sufficiently met and he was better regulated and less anxious. In fact, it was only when he started sensory integration therapy and his issues were addressed that he had begun to respond to his name, eventually developing his receptive and expressive language skills. The key, then, to opening up communication with dysregulated children was by addressing their sensory needs. Hence, the shift from a primarily psychodynamic stance to include a developmental one happened almost naturally, and I learned to use art materials for regulation purposes within the safe holding environment of the therapeutic relationship.

Eventually, what led me to the development of the Sensory-Based Relational Art Therapy Approach (S-BRATA) was the desire to seek a deeper understanding of an approach that I had developed organically over the years while working with children with autism and comorbid SID. The way I conducted art therapy seemed to work well for these children, but there were gaps in my knowledge that needed to be filled, and a doctorate seemed to be the best way to bridge those gaps between theory and practice.

S-BRATA is the result of the search for a deeper understanding of a concern that was instigated by my son's condition and gradually grew into a passion. Essentially, the framework that S-BRATA provides for doing art therapy with children with autism is preliminary; however, it has potential for further development and growth. Importantly, S-BRATA is not meant as a guide for art therapists alone but for all professionals using a multisensory kinesthetic approach, be it art, music, dance/movement or other therapies espousing a mind-body approach. Due to the flexibility of its scope and its capacity to integrate different modes of expression and creativity, the principles of the S-BRATA can be adapted and incorporated across multiple disciplines. The relational aspect of the S-BRATA can also serve as a guide for caregivers who want to gain insight into interacting and communicating with children with sensory challenges and those who may be highly anxious and appear to be averse to interaction with the outside world.

An Overview of the Chapters

Below is a brief introduction to the chapters of the book, which have been sequenced to illustrate the development of the study that led to the development of the S-BRATA.

Chapter 1 provides a brief history of autism and the traditional interventions that focus on behavior modification and skill building. It highlights the lack of focus on the psycho-emotional health of the child with autism that may not be prioritised over behavior management and teaching of skills. Next, it addresses caregiver stress related to raising a child with autism and associated behavioral and developmental challenges.

Chapter 2 explains attachment theory and SID. It underscores the significance of a healthy pattern of attachment for a child's emotional and developmental health and how the presence of SID may be playing a crucial role in the impairment of attachment patterns in children with autism.

Chapter 3 positions art therapy as an intervention that can concurrently address both attachment and sensory regulation in children with ASD due to its relational and sensorial aspects. It delineates current art therapy research and psychological theories that influenced the S-BRATA and its underlying themes and provides the rationale for the research that led to it.

Chapter 4 explicates the procedures and the methodology that led to the generation of the S-BRATA. It includes figures and tables that illustrate the grounded theory methodology that was used to develop the framework.

Chapter 5 to 11 detail the seven themes of the S-BRATA and their sub-themes, namely:

(1) Sense of Safety

    (a) holding back
    (b) making art yourself
    (c) approach, engage and retreat and
    (d) body positioning

(2) Sensory Regulation

    (a) observation and anticipation
    (b) practicing self-regulation and
    (c) being comfortable with unpredictability

(3) Mirroring and Attunement

    (a) rupture and repair
    (b) countertransference and self-awareness
    (c) body language and positioning and
    (d) tone of voice

(4) Art Materials as Entry Point For Engagement

    (a) the lure of art materials and
    (b) lack of motivation

(5) Structure and Boundaries;
(6) Flexibility

    (a) the space as a playground
    (b) toys, musical instruments and more and

(7) Art Product Not the Focus. Each theme is illustrated through case vignettes and related artwork.

Chapter 12 concludes with a summary of the S-BRATA. It briefly addresses topics such as self-care, supervision and response art and poses recommendations for future research and development of the framework.

The following terms are used interchangeably:

Autism spectrum disorder (ASD), autism, the spectrum
Child on the spectrum, child with autism spectrum disorder, child with autism, child, children
Caregiver, mother, parent
Art therapy studio, therapy room, room, studio
Shaving foam, foam

Part I

Autism, Attachment and Sensory Integration Dysfunction

1 Raising a Child on the Spectrum

A Brief History of ASD and Traditional Treatments

In 1943, a physician at John Hopkins University, Leo Kanner, was one of the first to identify autism or *infantile autism*, after observing children who shared a pattern of symptoms such as the need for sameness and solitude. Based on his observation, Kanner claimed that these children had "inborn autistic disturbances of affective contact," implying that they lacked the inherent ability to form relationships (Kanner, 1943, p. 250). Kanner initially leaned toward a biological explanation for autism because, according to him, these children appeared to exhibit their characteristic behaviors from an early age. Later, however, he changed his opinion to take in a psychological perspective that popularised the idea of autism as caused by inadequate parenting and used the term *refrigerator mothers* to characterise their inability to relate to their children with typical warmth and empathy (Kanner, 1943). The opinion that implicated poor parenting as the cause for autism was further popularised in 1967 by Bruno Bettelheim, an influential psychologist at the University of Chicago. Kanner's and Bettelheim's perspective guided the medical profession on autism for a quarter of a century (Grandin & Panek, 2013) and resulted in mothers blaming themselves for the condition of their child. Hans Asperger, who was Kanner's contemporary, published a paper in German in the 1940s describing a condition he called *autistic psychopathology* pertaining to children with restricted interests, rigid behaviors and inappropriate social relationships. Asperger's work was largely ignored, possibly because it was in German and maybe due to intellectual theft, only to receive recognition later when children with autism with strong intellectual ability and verbal language were classified as having Asperger's Syndrome (Silberman, 2015).

Subsequently, the disciplines of medicine and psychiatry evolved, and the definition and diagnosis of autism changed as the classification of psychiatric illnesses became more precise and ordered. For instance, autism had been confused with schizophrenia early on; the development of a diagnostic checklist of autistic behaviors that did not overlap with those of schizophrenia resulted in a formal diagnosis of the condition with its presenting criteria (Grandin & Panek, 2013).

Experts such as Bernard Rimland, a psychologist and parent of a child with autism; Lorna Wing, a psychiatrist; and Ivar Lovaas, a clinical psychologist contributed significantly toward the understanding and treatment of autism. Wing (1996) revived the work of Asperger and introduced the term *Asperger's Syndrome* to identify children on the higher functioning end of the spectrum. In fact, it is Wing (1996) who is credited for identifying autism as a spectrum rather than a differentiated disorder or disorders. Rimland (1964) refuted the myth of the refrigerator mother through his writing, based on observations of his own child, that he believed implicated a neural origin of autism. Rimland's opinion was widely welcomed by distraught parents who were being blamed for causing autism in their children.

Finally, by the 1990s and early 21st century, the human genome project revolutionised the study of genetics, and in 2007 specific areas of the genome were implicated in the etiology of autism (Grandin & Panek, 2013). Concurrently, a publication in the *Lancet* of a study that examined whether the measles, mumps and rubella (MMR) vaccine might be a cause of autism gained popularity as a theory among the general public (Wakefield, 1998). This theory continues to be contested as credible, even though the original research study that made a claim has been disproved (Deer, 2011).

Autism spectrum disorder (ASD) is now a singular diagnosis recognised as a continuum of comorbid difficulties with speech and language, social skills, psycho-motor regulation, sensory integration, theory of mind, restricted repetitive behaviors (RRBs) and self-stimulatory behaviors also known as *stimming*, among others (American Psychiatric Association, 2013). Autism is classified according to severity of scales (levels 1–3) depending on the level of support required for daily functioning, and the diagnosis of Asperger syndrome has been removed from the Diagnostic and Statistical Manual of Mental Disorders (DSM-5). For a diagnosis of autism, the symptoms must be present from an early age even though diagnosis occurs later in life.

According to the most recent statistics (Centres for Disease Control & Prevention, 2019) 1 in 59 children is diagnosed with autism, and boys are four times more likely than girls to have autism. While autism can be diagnosed as early as 2 years of age, most children receive a diagnosis around 4 years old. The prevalence of autism has resulted in a paradigm shift among the supporters of the neurodiversity movement who support the social model of viewing ASD as a natural variation of the human genome as opposed to the medical model that pathologises it as a disability. Champions of the neurodiversity movement denounce interventions that focus on changing autistic behaviors and looking for ways to fix autism. They advocate for accommodation and inclusion of individuals with differences without having to conform to the accepted standards of normality imposed by society.

Most treatments for ASD have focused primarily on modifying behaviors and the teaching of skills driven by the long term objective of enabling individuals with autism to achieve self-dependency. Below is a brief description of some of the traditional approaches that are available for caregivers to choose from once a diagnosis of autism has been made. The list is by no means complete or exhaustive; however, it is indicative of the trend toward targeting the behavioral, communication and skill building needs of the child with autism.

ABA

Lovaas (1987) pioneered the first behavioral intervention called Applied Behavior Analysis (ABA) which is based on the principles of operant conditioning that focus on teaching skills by breaking them into small steps and using a reward, punishment, reinforcement system. ABA is delivered as a one-on-one intensive treatment over 20–40 hours in the week. The progress of the child is recorded and reviewed regularly to make adjustments. ABA has evoked considerable controversy over the years because in its initial form, it was believed to be a harsh approach that punished unwanted behaviors. More recently, the proponents of the neurodiversity movement called the intervention an affront to individuals with autism as according to them it attempts to normalise a child with autism rather than accepting him or her as naturally different. Nevertheless, ABA, which is now available in modified versions such as the Pivotal Response Training (PRT), is the most scientifically researched of all autism specific interventions and continues to be a treatment of choice for many.

TEACCH

Treatment and Education of Autistic and Related Communication Handicapped Children (TEACCH) was developed in the 1970s to target specific social, communication and developmental needs of the child. TEACCH is a highly structured approach that is conducted in an environment modified to accommodate the child.

RDI

Relationship Development Intervention (RDI) focuses on the parent- child relationship by training the parents through intensive workshops and videos. The goal of the therapy is the social development of the child with autism.

DIR *Floortime*

Dr. Stanely Greenspan (2002), a psychiatrist, pioneered the Developmental, Individual-Difference, Relationship Based (DIR) Floortime approach, which, as its name suggests, encourages the caregiver or therapist to get on the floor and interact with the child in an unstructured, playful manner. The goal of the intervention is to build an attachment with the therapist or caregiver by increasing the circles of communication with the child through following the lead of the child.

OT, Speech and Language Therapy (Splt) and Others

Apart from the autism specific interventions described above, most children require some degree of occupational therapy (OT) for psychomotor challenges and sensory integration and speech and language therapy to address language and communication issues. Recently, nutritional interventions that may include a diet of essential fatty acids, a healthy gluten-free, casein-free, soy-free (HGCSF) diet and vitamin/mineral supplements, have gained traction due to evidence of nutritional deficiencies, metabolic and digestive imbalances in children with autism (Adams et al., 2018).

I, too, opted for the most popular interventions for ASD for Moeez soon after he was diagnosed. For the first few years, Moeez's regimen consisted of OT, TEACCH, and Splt apart from the playschool he attended. Lured by the promise of progress, I delved into alternative treatments like cranio-sacral therapy and homeopathy, switching from TEACCH to ABA when Moeez turned 8 years old. After Moeez entered double digits, he was weaned off ABA but continued with OT and intermittent Splt with decreasing frequency. In his teens, he received counseling as and when the need arose. While Moeez was growing up, art therapy was a very new and almost unknown profession in Singapore; hence, he was not able to avail its benefits. Moreover, my primary focus had been managing Moeez's behaviors and teaching him life skills, like most other caregivers.

Challenges for Caregivers

Research shows that caregivers of children with autism experience higher levels of stress, anxiety and depression than those of typically developing children as well as children with disabilities other than autism (Fernell, Eriksson, & Gilberg, 2013; Teague, Newman, Tonge, & Gray, 2018). The stress emanates from challenging behaviors that are found to be more prevalent in children on the spectrum than in children with other intellectual and developmental differences. The behaviors may include acute tantrums, acts of aggression or self-harm toward self or others and socially unacceptable behaviors (Ang & Loh, 2019) as well as "children's disturbed sleep, agitation and cries, stereotypy and self-injury, difficulties in feeding and toilet training, epileptic seizures, lack of social or emotional reciprocity and other unusual behaviours" (Cappe, Wolff, Bobet, & Adrien, 2011). The severity of symptoms/behaviors in the children and degree of functional independence are correlated to the frequency of mental health issues in caregivers. Lack of social and emotional support and criticism from the community about certain behaviors may add to the anxiety of caregivers who are already dealing with multiple pressures at home. Benson and Karlof (2008) cite *stress proliferation* as another factor that may contribute to the stress of caregivers. Stress proliferation refers to primary and secondary stressors that act on each other to create additional stress resulting in psychological distress. For instance, sustained caregiving of a child with severe ASD (primary stressor) may translate into financial stress (secondary stressor) and so on. Referring to a study conducted by Benson (2006), the authors posit that stress proliferation is a strong predictor of self-reported depression in caregivers correlated to the severity of symptoms of autism. "The challenges in identifying, accessing, and paying for ASD services, given the nature of these children's needs, available resources, and complex financing arrangements, can place a substantial burden on caregivers" (Cohrs & Leslie, 2017, p. 1416).

I recall several occasions with Moeez, especially when he was nonverbal, where a tantrum would emerge out of nowhere in the middle of a shopping mall triggered by some demand that he was unable to communicate. Although I was never an apologetic or embarrassed parent, these incidents were nevertheless stress inducing since they were unpredictable and difficult to manage. In Moeez's younger days, visits to the barber for a haircut were often accompanied by behaviors such as involuntary laughter or singing that were a source of embarrassment to his younger brother who was learning to live with a differently abled older sibling. One particular incident still stands out in my memory as a traumatic event with respect to societal ignorance and lack of acceptance, when a woman openly threatened 12-year-old Moeez in a mall for accidentally backing his scooter on her ankle. She continued to rant at him even after she was told that he had autism and he had profusely apologised for his error. Societal expectations and lack of understanding in the larger community continue to present occasional challenges for Moeez, especially since he has grown into a young questioning adult with his own worldview.

All caregivers respond differently to the stress of raising a differently abled child. Their response depends upon their style of coping, adaptation, quality of life, social and emotional support (Vogan et al., 2014). Lai and Oei (2014) assert there are positive and negative coping strategies that are predictors of mental health outcomes. Carver (1997) identified the following coping strategies that are applicable to caregivers of children on the spectrum (Ang & Loh, 2019).

Active avoidance: escaping from facing the problem and using emotion-driven strategies; resorting to substance abuse, disengagement and self-blame.

Problem focused coping: actively addressing the stressors by seeking social-emotional support and looking for solutions.

Positive: recontextualising the problem through acceptance and positive outlook; seeking social-emotional support.

Religious/denial coping: resorting to prayer and spiritual means or refusal to accept.

Lai and Oei (2014) brought attention to cultural differences that can impact coping strategies across the globe. Citing different world views of the East (collectivism) and West (individualism) as possible influences on approach and outcomes, they asserted that "there is possibility of a degree of mitigated risk for psychological maladjustment among Asian parents of children with ASD as compared to western European parents" (p. 2). However, they add that Asian caregivers may put more emphasis on academic achievement and avoid talking about their problems to *save face*, which may contribute to increased stress.

The Oversight That May Be Happening

Most caregivers of a newly diagnosed child with autism are blown away by the shock of the diagnosis of ASD and its implications. Coming to terms with the diagnosis is often a journey involving denial, anger, depression and acceptance. Emotional turmoil aside, caregivers are bombarded with a choice of interventions – some traditionally used for autism and some alternative ones that may have benefitted others. Typically, a child diagnosed with autism would have speech and language therapy, OT as well as one of the behavior focused treatments mentioned above. The plate of the child as well as the caregiver is often very full with the therapeutic regimen of the child, together with the demands of the school the child may be attending. Hence, a therapeutic approach that targets unwanted behaviors would be a natural first choice, followed by development of communication skills and life skills. As noted earlier, the daunting task of cognizant parenting of a child with ASD may overwhelm the most capable of caregivers.

It was only during my Master's program in art therapy that I realised that I had taken Moeez's emotional well-being for granted. I had assumed that since he had grown up with a loving and supportive family, his psycho-emotional needs had been met. Moeez presented as a happy child in general, barring periods of extreme anxiety where the stimming and RRBs would escalate. Although Moeez was verbal, he struggled to understand his emotions and express them. Facilitating his expression would have possibly lessened his anxiety and enhanced his mental health.

The fact that the emotional well-being of the child with autism can get passed over due to the emphasis on behavior modification and the teaching of skills hit home especially when I worked with nonverbal children who had very limited means of expression. Whereas Moeez had functional communication, some of my clients were highly anxious, and their only means of expression were behaviors that were often a source of distress for their caregivers. One such child was 12-year-old Nathan (psuedonym) who had autism, was nonverbal and had difficulty walking due to cerebral palsy that had affected his limbs. Nathan received OT, speech therapy and physiotherapy when he came to me for art therapy soon after I began practicing. He was well built and very strong for his age, which made handling him difficult especially when he indulged in self-harm and aggressive behaviors toward others. Nathan's parents were distraught as nothing seemed to calm him down, and most other therapists were reluctant to work with him. As a novice art therapist, I, too, struggled with Nathan's behaviors and found it extremely challenging to motivate him. Nevertheless, taking it up as a challenge, I worked with Nathan for about a year before I had to stop because I was leaving Singapore for a few years. In retrospect, I wonder how much of Nathan's defiance and volatility was a symptom of years of pent up frustration he was unable to express or channel in an appropriate manner. Undoubtedly, children like Nathan require interventions that teach them life skills and adaptive behaviors, but it is critical not to ignore the feeling, sensing child who is often trapped inside a recalcitrant body.

Talking of children's emotional well-being, one of the fundamental building blocks of children's psycho-emotional health is their first relationship, also known as the attachment relationship with their caregiver. The attachment pattern of a child lays the blueprint of his or her future relationships and has long term implications for mental well-being. For children with autism who have inherent relational and communication challenges, the importance of the attachment relationship cannot be emphasised enough. Spurred by my personal and professional interest in the mental health of children with autism, I was drawn to look deeper into attachment within the context of ASD.

A Rising Concern

Moeez was my first child and I aspired to be his best possible caregiver. Therefore, when Moeez refused to latch on to my breast to feed, I chided myself for my inexperience. After considerable effort, Moeez finally latched on, but what should have been a pleasurable experience for him seemed to evoke the opposite reaction. Baffled by Moeez's crying and apparent distress, I was left feeling helpless and guilty. Rather than risk starving my child, I switched to the bottle, to which Moeez took instantly. According to Slade (2009), "With children on the spectrum, the signposts that ordinarily help parents make sense of their child's inner experiences, such as eye contact, typical indicators of pleasure, pain, fear and sadness, directed communication, and the like are missing or disrupted" (p. 10). What I had misconstrued as my failure to breastfeed my child was in reality my inability to understand the reason of his displeasure, a possible result of oral sensitivity. Feeding from the breast required considerably more effort than sucking milk from the bottle, which may have exacerbated Moeez's oral discomfort and subsequent resistance to breast feeding. Consequently, one of my first attempts to synch emotionally and psychologically with my son was hampered by sensory challenges that I would only become aware of after his diagnosis of ASD.

Later in life, I began to question my attachment pattern with Moeez, especially when I delved deeper into attachment theory. Even though I believed I was a *secure base* for my child since he sought comfort and proximity to me, I extrapolated that there was a possibility of qualitative differences between the attachment patterns of neurotypical children on the spectrum due to the presence of sensory issues. Further research into attachment theory within the context of autism confirmed my suspicions.

Conclusion

ASD is a complex condition that affects the individual on the spectrum across neurobiological, psycho-emotional, developmental and behavioral domains. The comorbidities that are inherent in the spectrum can make life extremely challenging for the child with autism, instigating behaviors that are difficult to manage and a source of anguish for his or her caregivers. Behavior focused interventions may be prioritised by caregivers to address taxing behaviors. The psycho-emotional well-being of the child with autism can be passed over when the focus is on the teaching of skills and behavior management. Caregivers for children with ASD report a high instance of mental health issues that arise from the stress of caregiving and correlated stressors. A healthy attachment pattern with the primary caregiver plays a critical role in the healthy psycho-emotional development of a child and has implications for the emotional health of a child with autism.

References

Adams, B. J., Audhya, T., Geis, A., Gehn, E., Fimbres, V., Pollard, L. E., & Quig, W. D. (2018). Comprehensive nutritional and dietary intervention for autism spectrum disorder—A randomized, controlled 12-month trial. *Nutrients, 10*(3), 369. https://doi.org/10.3390/nu10030369.

American Psychiatric Association. (2013). *Diagnostic and statistical manual of mental disorders* (5th ed.). Washington, DC: Author.

Ang, P. Q. K., & Loh, R. P. (2019). Mental health and coping in parents of children with autism spectrum disorder (ASD) in Singapore: An examination of gender role in caring. *Journal of Autism and Developmental Disorders, 49*, 2129–2145. https://doi.org/10.1007/s10803-019-03900-w.

Benson, P. R. (2006). The impact of symptom severity of depressed mood among parents of children with ASD: The mediating role of stress proliferation. *Journal of Autism and Developmental Disorders, 36*, 685–695. 10.1007/s10803-006-0112-3.

Benson, P. R., & Karlof, L. K. (2008). Anger, stress proliferation, and depressed mood among parents of children with ASD: A longitudinal replication. *Journal of Autism and Developmental Disorders, 39*, 350–362. 10.1007/s10803-008-0632-0.

Cappe, E., Wolff, M., Bobet, R., & Adrien, J. L. (2011). Quality of life: A key variable to consider in the evaluation of adjustment in parents of children with autism spectrum disorders and in the development of relevant support and assistance programmes. *Quality of Life Research, 20*, 1279–1294. 10.1007/s11136-011-9861-3.

Carver, C. S. (1997). You want to measure coping but your protocol's too long: Consider the brief COPE. *International Journal of Behavioral Medicine, 4*(1), 92–100.

Centers for Disease Control & Prevention (Sept. 19, 2019). Retrieved from https://www.cdc.gov/ncbddd/autism/data.html.

Cohrs, C. A., & Leslie, L. D. (2017). Depression in parents of children diagnosed with autism spectrum disorder: A claims-based analysis. *Journal of Autism and Developmental Disorders, 47*, 1416–1422. 10.1007/s10803-017-3063-y.

Deer, B. (2011). How the case against the MMR vaccine was fixed. *BMJ, 342*, c5347–c5347. 10.1136/bmj.c5347.

Fernell, E., Eriksson, A. M., & Gilberg, C. (2013). Early diagnosis of autism and impact on prognosis: A narrative review. *Clinical Epidemiology, 5,* 33–43.

Grandin, T., & Panek, R. (2013). *The autistic brain.* New York, NY: Houghton Mifflin Harcourt.

Greenspan, S. I. (2002). *The secure child: Helping our children feel safe and confident in a changing world.* Cambridge, MA: Da Capo Press.

Kanner, L. (1943). Autistic disturbances of affective contact. *Nervous Child, 2,* 217–250.

Lai, W. W., & Oei, S. P. T. (2014). Coping in parents and caregivers of children with autism spectrum disorders (ASD): A review. *Review Journal of Autism and Developmental Disorders, 1,* 207–224. 10.1007/s40489-014-0021-x.

Lovaas, O. I. (1981). *Teaching developmentally disabled children: The me book.* Baltimore, MD: University Park Press.

Lovaas, O. I. (1987). Behavioral treatment and normal educational and intellectual functioning in young autistic children. *Journal of Consulting and Clinical Psychology, 55,* 3–9.

Rimland, B. (1964). *Infantile autism: The syndrome and its implications for a neural theory of behavior.* East Norwalk, CT, US: Appleton-Century-Crofts.

Silberman, S. (2015). *Neurotribes: The legacy of autism and the future of neurodiversity.* New York, NY: Avery.

Slade, A. (2009). Metalizing the unmentalizable: Parenting children on the spectrum. *Journal of Infant, Child and Adolescent Psychotherapy, 8*(1), 7–21. 10.1080/15289160802683054.

Teague, J. S., Newman, K. L., Tonge, J. B., & Gray, M. K. (2018). Caregiver mental health, parenting practices, and perceptions of child attachment in children with autism spectrum disorder. *Journal of Autism and Developmental Disorders, 48,* 2642–2652. https://doi.org/10.1007/s10803-018-3517-x.

Vogan, V., Lake, K. J., Weiss, A. J., Robinson, S., Tint, A., & Lunsky, Y. (2014). Factors associated with caregiver burden am parents of individuals with ASD: Differences across intellectual functioning. *Family Relations, 63,* 554–567. doi:10.1111/fare.12081.

Wakefield, A. J. (1998). MMR vaccination and autism. *Lancet, 354*(9182), 949–950.

Wing, L. (1996). *The autistic spectrum.* London, UK: Constable and Company Ltd.

2 Attachment and Sensory Integration Dysfunction (SID)

Bowlby's (1969) attachment theory drew from mid 20th century Western ethology (i.e., the study of animal behavior to understand humans) and comparative psychology at a time when significant advances in knowledge were being made in biology. He elucidated that human infants are born with an innate desire to attach to other humans and that this desire to connect with others is the result of the process of natural selection or evolution. Stern (1977) elaborated that attachment, also known as the first relationship, is rooted in certain behaviors between caregiver and child; he called this reciprocal exchange "the choreography of maternal behaviors" (p. 23). The behavior that Stern referred to may be compared to a dance between two partners – the caregiver, the leading partner, matching the affective state of the child in intensity and duration while teaching the child the steps of the dance (Hughes, 2004). An analogy may also be drawn to a scenario of a mother responding to her infant's cry for milk. The mother, while preparing the milk bottle for the infant, may shake a rattle in one hand to divert the child's attention. By performing these two acts instinctively, not only does she gratify the infant's hunger, she also regulates him by diverting his focus from a painful stimulus to a positive one. In turn, the child stops crying at the sound and sight of the rattle and once he starts feeding, he rewards his mother by gazing lovingly into her eyes. Consistent modeling of such behaviors by the mother and consonant responses of the child over time lay the foundation of an attachment pattern through which the child learns to understand the world and deal with it effectively. The two-way explicit and implicit communication between caregiver and child is mediated through attachment behaviors like eye gaze, vocalisations such as cooing, hand gestures, touch and multiple nuanced interactions that are the gateway to the psychological, emotional and social bonding between them.

Bowlby's attachment theory emphasised the criticality of a child's early life experiences as having long-term implications for mental and developmental health (as cited in Sroufe, Carlson, Levy, & Egeland, 1999). Building on Bowlby's theory, current research affirms that the attachment relationship is correlated to a sense of security, resilience and the ability to self-soothe in the child. Securely attached children learn to trust themselves and others and can seek support from others when in need of emotional regulation (Shaver & Mikulinger, 2002; Shore, 2014). van der Kolk (2014) reiterated that self-regulation is dependent to no small degree on harmonious relations with the caregiver; children learn that others have feelings similar and different from them through the reciprocity of attachment. From their earliest life experiences onward, the synchrony of the mother-child relationship or attunement gives infants the sense that their needs are being met. Hence, a healthy first relationship between caregiver and child is likely to contribute significantly to the latter's psycho-emotional development and mental health.

Though it is not within the scope of this book to address the universality of attachment theory, it is pertinent to mention that some researchers question the validity of the theory across cultures since it is rooted in mainstream Western psychology (Rothbaum, Weisz, Pott, Miyake, & Morelli, 2000).

Types of Attachment

Attachment may be classified as organised and disorganised. Organised type attachment may be further categorised as secure, insecure avoidant and insecure resistant, and disorganised type attachment as insecure disorganised (Benoit, 2004). An attachment pattern begins to take shape when the infant, at around 6 months of age, starts to anticipate the caregiver's response to his or her distress and reacts accordingly. An infant is likely to develop a secure attachment when met regularly with a sensitive and loving response from a caregiver. Consequently, an organised pattern of seeking proximity to the caregiver is established when assured of a consistently sensitive response. Where the caregiver responds insensitively to the infant, the latter learns to avoid interaction and subdue his or her emotions, resulting in an organised but avoidant pattern of rejection of the caregiver in times of distress. Similarly, an insecure resistant pattern emerges from unpredictable caregiving where inconsistent responses toward the infant exact extreme attention-seeking behaviors from the latter. The children who do not follow any of the above organised strategies or responses fall under the insecure disorganised type of attachment pattern.

Hughes (2004) described attachment patterns within the context of a child's typical developmental stages. He identified the following six attachment stages and the developmental milestones correlating to them, spanning the period of a child's first 4 years of life (see Table 2.1).

Attachment in Children with ASD

Kanner's initial definition of autism led to the misconception that children on the spectrum did not have the innate ability to form attachment relationships. This was followed by another fallacy that implicated poor parenting for causing autism in children. Subsequent studies employing clinical observation have verified that children with autism do show attachment behavior (Buitelaar,

Homeostatis/Concrete Attachment (0-3months)	Indiscriminate attachment; increased interest in external stimuli; attempts at self-regulation
Attachment/Personal Attachment (0-7months)	Attention directed towards specific caregiver; emotional involvement and synchrony with caregiver; responsive to caregiver's touch and smile
Somatopsychological Differentiation/Intentional Attachment (3-10months)	Purposeful attachment; reciprocity; interaction based on cause and effect
Behavioral Organization/Conceptual and Integrated Attachment (9-18 months)	Organized emotional responses, increased range of meaningful behaviors; interaction and separation
Representational Capacity/InternalSymbolic Attachment (18-30 months)	Emergence of language to communicate desire and feelings
Representational Differentiation/Differentiated Attachments (24-48months)	Wider range of emotions; concept of separation between self and others

Table 2.1 Stages of attachment development

1995; Rogers, Ozonoff, & Maslin-Cole, 1993). These studies were based on the Strange Situation Procedure (SSP) that measures attachment in neurotypical children. Observation of attachment in children with autism became more accurate when the SSP was modified and carried out in the more naturalistic and less stressful environment of the child's home through the Attachment Q Sort (Rutgers, Van Ijzendoorn, Bakermans-Kranenburg, & Swinkles, 2007; Vaughn & Waters, 1990). The Attachment Q Sort was developed by Waters and Deane (1985) as an alternative to the SSP. The SSP can only be conducted once on children in their second year, restricting it to a specific period of attachment development, and its ethical validity is questioned due to the stress-inducing separation episode that is conducted in an artificial clinical environment (Van Ijzendoorn, Vereijken, Bakersman-Kranenberg, & Riksen-Walraven, 2004). The Attachment Q sort, on the other hand, has, among other advantages over the SSP, the scope to measure a broader age range from

1 to 4 years of age and may be conducted multiple times with the same child. It has higher ecological validity as it can be administered at home, does not require the stressful separation behavior and is culturally sensitive (Van Ijzendoorn et al., 2004). In fact, a meta-analytic review of studies of children with autism that measured attachment via modified SSPs (Rutgers et al., 2007) confirmed evidence of attachment behaviors in children with autism such as preference for a specific caregiver and anxiety at unexpected separation from them (Rogers, Ozonoff, & Maslin-Cole, 1991) while acknowledging that the pattern of attachment may be less secure than that of typical children (Ainsworth, Blehar, Waters, & Wall, 1978; Rutgers et al., 2007). A more recent review by Teague, Newman, Tonge, and Gray (2018) found that only 47% of children with autism were securely attached. According to Rutgers et al. (2007), the quality of attachment in children with autism appears to be less attuned and flexible and there is less display of reciprocal attachment behaviors such as smiling, playing and frequent looking.

Unfortunately, there is scant research on impaired or disorganised attachment in children with autism, and the studies that exist were mostly conducted on children older than 3 years of age (Naber et al., 2007) when the optimum period for attachment has already passed. However, researchers have hypothesised various probable reasons of impaired attachment.

Taking into account the importance of reciprocal communication in the formation of an attachment, it makes sense that the following differences in children with autism compared to neurotypical children would play a critical role in its quality.

Baron-Cohen (1989) and Stern (1985) pointed to developmental delays in children with ASD, Naber et al. (2007) implicated cognitive differences, whereas other researchers (e.g., Sivaratnam, Newman, Tonge, & Rinehart, 2015) cite differences in social and emotional development. Children who are 12 months and older with high risk of autism have been observed to have less joint attention (ability to share focus on an object with another person) (Presmanes, Walden, Stone, & Yoder, 2007) and decreased social communication and responses to their name (Nadig et al., 2007) and reward cues (Garon et al., 2009). Consider as an example the case of joint attention and its implications on relational development between a child with autism and the caregiver. When the child is unable to share an interest in an object with another individual, the caregiver's attempts to direct the child toward environmental stimuli would possibly go unnoticed. This lack of joint attention would adversely affect the exchange of verbal and nonverbal communication and, consequently, the pattern of attachment between the two subjects.

Further to the findings cited above, Beurkens, Hobson, and Hobson (2013) noted that very young children with autism have "impairments in the frequency or intensity of eye contact, turn-taking, and referential looking" (p. 169). Klin, Lin, Gorrindo, Ramsay, and Jones (2009) found evidence that children with ASD may pay more attention to non-social or physical contingencies than to movements that signal social cues such as facial expressions and gaze direction. In contrast, preferential attention to social cues is integral to the development of relationships and the attribution of intention to others, both of which are central features of forming an attachment with the caregiver. If, as the authors contended, the child with autism does not pay as much attention to the face and gaze of the caregiver, then a fundamental attachment behavior is taken out of the equation of reciprocity between the two. This social and developmental difference has many implications for mutual co-regulation and attunement achieved through the gaze, facial expressions and gestures of the caregiver aimed at the child (Schore, 2003). Emery (2002) added that children who cannot relate to people "go through infancy without acquiring a concept of persons as subjects of experience ... any sensory deprivation can limit a child's experience and, therefore, alter his or her behaviors" (p. 144).

While some researchers have investigated attachment in children with ASD through the lens of development issues and social and emotional behaviors, others such as Ben-Sasson et al. (2007) considered the quality of attachment concerning sensory regulation issues. High arousal, psychological stress and anxiety occur in children who have difficulty integrating incoming sensory information from the environment. These sensory regulation issues that cause atypical processing of auditory, visual and tactile stimuli result in the impairment of learning that comes from people and the world around them (Marco, Hinkley, Hill, & Nagarajan, 2011). Imagine an infant who is extremely sensitive to sound or hyposensitive to touch. Attempts at physical affection by the caregiver might be rejected out of protection from pain, as would touching unfamiliar things in the environment; such avoidance over time puts relational and developmental learning at risk for the child with ASD.

There is an increasing body of evidence that shows that a healthy attachment has positive psycho-emotional and developmental outcomes for children with autism (Teague et al., 2018). Given the immense challenges that children with autism face in the communication, social, emotional and sensory domains, it is all the more pertinent to understand the mutuality that goes into forming a healthy attachment. It is especially necessary to consider the impact of SID on impaired attachment in children with ASD, considering that it can affect multiple channels of communication across the senses.

Sensory Integration Dysfunction (SID)

> YOU KNOW WHAT I HATE? The sound of hand dryers in public restrooms. Not so much when the air jet starts, but the moment someone's hand enter the stream. The sudden drop in register drives me nuts. It's like when the vacuum toilet on an airplane flushes. First comes the brief rain like prelude, then a thunderclap of suction. I *hate* that. *Fingernails-on-a-chalk board* hate.
>
> (Temple Grandin)

Hyper-responsiveness	Over-reaction to stimuli, examples include aversion to touch and texture such as labels on clothes, dislike of hugs, refusal to walk barefoot on grass, awareness of smells and sounds that may lead to sensory overload.
Hypo-responsiveness or sensory gating	Under-reaction to stimuli, for example, diminished response to extremely hot and cold surfaces, disengagement from environment, not responding to name being called etc.
Sensory seeking	Seeking extreme stimulation, for example enjoy rough play, touching and sniffing objects, excessive fidgeting, swinging etc.
Sensory defensive	Negative reaction to sensory input. Child is hyper-responsive to sensory stimuli and protects themselves through negative reaction.
Sensory avoidant	Resistance to interact with environment due to over-response to sensory stimuli.

Table 2.2 Commonly used terms in sensory processing

When the brain is unable to process sensory information from the environment optimally and the pattern consistently disrupts the emotional, behavioral and motor functioning of the child, it is classified as a disorder or SID. SID, otherwise also known as sensory processing disorder, can affect any of the sensory domains of vision, auditory, kinesthetic, taste, smell, vestibular (sense of movement) and proprioception (sense of body in space) (Marco et al., 2011).

Hilton et al. (2010) contended that, generally speaking, there are three types of sensory modulation issues: sensory under-responsiveness, sensory over-responsiveness and sensory seeking (i.e., actively seeking and engaging with stimuli). A child could be hypo- and hypersensitive in any of the sensory domains at the same time (see Table 2.2). For instance, a child with auditory hypersensitivity may find certain everyday sounds, like the running of a tap, unbearable, whereas the same child could be hyposensitive to sound and may not respond to being called by his name. Referring to her challenges with sensory over-responsiveness, Temple Grandin described why she was unable to be physically affectionate toward her mother, stating, "The problem, though, wasn't that I did not want her. It was that the sensory overload of a hug shorted out my nervous system" (Grandin & Panek, 2013, p. 8).

As mentioned earlier, Moeez had extreme sensory challenges in the proprioceptive domain. The lying down behavior or stim was a manifestation of his need to feel his body parts through contact with the floor. However, proprioception was not his only sensory modality that was affected, it was only the most obvious one because of its severity. Moeez also had some visual and auditory impairments, the former causing him to stim with objects he jiggled close to his eyes and the latter giving rise to occasional outbursts, for example, when the sound of a running tap would be a source of great anxiety to him. Over time, Moeez's sensory needs fluctuated in prevalence. For instance, the proprioceptive stim reduced significantly, whereas the visual stim gained dominance. Over all, as Moeez grew past his teens, the frequency of his stimming patterns was reduced possibly because his sensory needs abated and he learned to self-regulate through other means.

Leekman, Nieto, Libby, Wing, and Gould (2007) examined the frequency and patterns of sensory abnormalities in children and adults with autism through two studies employing the Diagnostic Interview for Social and Communication Disorders. The first study compared children with autism and those without autism, whereas the follow-up study was more extensive and detailed, consisting of 200 individuals with autism, adults as well as children. Taken together, the researchers found that sensory deficits are distributed along an entire spectrum and do not follow a specific pattern; that is, some people with autism may have problems with audio-visual processing, whereas others may have challenges with proprioception, vestibulation or other singular or multiple sensory domains. Each individual with ASD has a unique sensory profile. Marco et al. (2011) reported that 96% of children with autism have difficult with sensory integration across diverse domains.

SID: A Probable Cause for Impaired Attachment in Children with Autism

Sensory regulation issues that cause atypical processing of auditory, visual and tactile stimuli result in the impairment of learning that comes from people and the world around them (Ben-Sasson et al., 2007; Marco et al., 2011). Imagine an infant who is extremely sensitive to sound or hyposensitive to touch. Attempts at physical affection by the caregiver might be rejected out of protection from pain, as would touching unfamiliar things in the environment; such avoidance over time puts relational and developmental learning at risk for the ASD child. Most attachment behaviors are experienced through sensory channels, and it follows that a disturbance in the sensory system will impact attachment formation.

Taking into account the importance of reciprocal communication in the formation of an attachment, it makes sense that the presence of SID would play a critical role in its quality.

Gomez and Baird (2005) noted that self-regulatory issues are present in children with autism from as early as 1 year of age. Although the authors did not specify the source of these regulatory challenges, Miller, Anzalone, Lane, Cermak, and Osten (2007) suggested that difficulty in organising and assimilating incoming sensory information from the environment may be a cause of dysregulation in children with ASD. Naber et al. (2007) correlated the presence of sensory challenges to anxiety in children with autism, whereas Ben-Sasson et al. reported a high incidence of depression and withdrawal.

I mentioned my struggle with breast feeding Moeez as an infant. I also recall how I thought he was an exceptionally happy infant, who, apart from feeding issues and recurrent croup (respiratory infection), rarely cried. I attributed Moeez's difficulty in falling asleep to an inherent predisposition and it never crossed my mind that the absence of mouthing behaviors (putting toys into the mouth to explore) could be the result of oral sensitivity. Gesturing and cooing behaviors that are the cornerstone of a mother-child relationship were completely absent between Moeez and me, and being a first time mother, I was oblivious to their significance. After I had my second child, who is neurotypical, the contrast of my experience between him and Moeez became very obvious. When I took up the issue with paediatricians in Pakistan, they brushed aside my concerns, and it was not until I moved to Singapore that Moeez was finally diagnosed. Even though some of the typical attachment behaviors such as vocalisations, gesturing and other nuanced interactions were missing between us, Moeez was able to form an attachment with me and I believe I was his secure base. In this context, one of the examples that particularly stands out is where, after Moeez started attending preschool, the first thing he would do after returning home would be to lie down in my lap with his milk bottle and caress my face with his free hand until he had finished drinking. Another one is bedtime, where he would snuggle close to me and only go to sleep if one of his hands was under my cheek. As Moeez grew older, these behaviors transformed into frequent hugs and seeking more and more emotional support as his self-awareness increased. Nevertheless, I am inclined to believe that the quality of his attachment was different from that of typical children and his SID probably had a major role to play.

According to van der Kolk (2014), without an integration of sensory experience, one cannot be "in synch with oneself and with others" (p. 124). This is particularly the case in early life when the infant's sensory apparatus is the dominant channel for meaning making and communication with the surrounding world as the higher brain or neocortical functions that deal with planning, rational and abstract thought mature later in the second year of life (van der Kolk, 2014). Conversely, the infant's limbic system, also sometimes referred to as the reptilian brain or the seat of emotions such pain, pleasure and fear, is first to develop immediately after birth and is experience dependent. Since the infant's sphere of experience in the first year of life is limited to a primarily sensorial world, it follows that a dysfunction in the sensory system that processes and integrates the sensations from the environment will have a direct impact on the emotional well-being of the child. Take, for example, an infant who may avoid eye contact as well as touch from the caregiver due to sensory challenges in the visual and tactile domains. Consequently, two of the primary attachment behaviors of eye gaze and touch would be compromised between caregiver and child, plausibly hampering optimal attachment.

Researchers have begun to identify the multiple domains and diverse sensory challenges that may be unique to each individual with autism. For instance, Sabatos-De Vito, Schipul, Bulluck, Belger, and Baranek (2016) noted deficits in the area of attention control and the ability to select, orient, engage and disengage from visual stimuli that may impact the social skills and sensory responses of children on the spectrum as well as encourage perseverative behaviors and restricted interests.

Conversely, Tomchek and Dunn (2007) documented visual processing differences such as avoidance of eye contact and ineffectual eye gaze that may be coping strategies to deal with difficulties in modulating incoming visual information. Hirstein, Iversen, and Ramachandran (2001) observed the tendency in the population with ASD to focus on objects atypically, including the use of peripheral vision for activities, unlike typical people who use focal vision. Tomchek and Dunn (2007) posited that auditory processing is the most common sensory issue in individuals with autism. Children with auditory processing difficulties may appear to be deaf when in reality they may shut down their auditory channels to block out sounds from the environment that may cause them extreme discomfort or pain (Wing, 1996).

Robledo, Donnellan, and Strand-Conroy (2012) documented self-stories told by individuals on the spectrum that reveal a wide range of unique sensory challenges and give insight into these trying experiences that Grandin referred to as an "alternate sensory reality" (Grandin & Panek 2013, p. 70). For instance, one person reported how she was able to listen better to someone speaking to her if she did not have to look them in the eye. She found it distracting to do so, causing her to lose focus and be unable to process what was being said to her. She added that particular sounds triggered painful emotions that made her lose control in front of other people. Another individual shared that she would often get stuck with certain words or phrases when trying to form and say a particular sentence. Something completely different than what she intended would come out instead; her mouth refused to listen to her mind. Most of these self-stories revealed significant challenges in the area of communication, emotional expression and psychomotor regulation in the context of relationships.

Conclusion

SID is a core symptom of ASD and is present in varying degrees, across multiple sensory domains in the majority of children with autism. SID which is known to cause dysregulation and anxiety in children on the spectrum, negatively impacts attachment behaviors between caregiver and child and may contribute to impaired attachment in them. Fortunately, attachment patterns are not set in stone and can be acquired later in life. Therefore, a healthy attachment subsequent to an impaired one can ameliorate the loss that the earlier, impaired attachment may have caused (Siegel, 2003). This discovery has positive implications for the treatment of impaired attachment in children with autism and necessitates the inclusion of an intervention in the child's therapeutic regimen that can tackle both SID and attachment concurrently.

References

Ainsworth, M. S., Blehar, M. S., Waters, E., & Wall, S. (1978). *Patterns of attachment: A psychological study of the strange situation.* New York, NY: Erlbaum.

American Psychiatric Association. (2013). *Diagnostic and statistical manual of mental disorders* (5th ed.). Washington, DC: Author.

Baron-Cohen, S. (1989). The autistic child's theory of mind: The case of specific developmental delay. *Journal of Clinical Child Psychology and Psychiatry, 30*(2), 285–298. 10.1111/j.1469-7610.1989.tb00241.x.

Benoit, D. (2004). Infant-parent attachment: Definition, types, antecedents,measurement and outcome. *Paediatrics & Child Health, 9*(8), 5545. https://doi.org/10.1093/pch/9.8.541.

Ben-Sasson, A., Cermak, S. A., Orsmond, G. I., Tager-Flusberg, H., Carter, A. S., Kadlec, M.B., & Dunn, W. (2007). Extreme snsory modulation behaviors in toddlers with autism spectrum disorders. *American Journal of Occupational Therapy, 61*(5), 584–592.

Beurkens, M. N., Hobson, A. J., & Hobson, P. R. (2013). Autism severity and qualities of parent-child relations. *Journal of Autism Development Disorder, 43*(1), 168–178. 10.1007/s10803-012-1562-4.

Bowlby, J. (1969). *Attachment and loss, Vol. 1: Attachment.* New York, NY: Basic Books.

Buitelaar, J. K. (1995). Attachment and social withdrawal in autism: Hypothesis and findings. *Behaviour, 132*(5), 319–350.

Emery, J. M. (2002). Art therapy as an intervention for autism. *Journal of the American Art Therapy Association, 2*(3), 143–147.

Garon, N., Bryson, S. E., Zwaigenbaum, L., Smith, I. M., Brian, J., Roberts, W., & Szatmari, P. (2009). Temperament and its relationship to autistic symptoms in a high-risk infant sib cohort. *Journal of Abnormal Child Psychology, 37*(1), 59–78. 10.1007/s10802-008-9258-0.

Gomez, C. R., & Baird, S. (2005). Identifying early indicators for autism in self-regulation difficulties. *Focus on Autism and Other Developmental Disabilities, 20*(2), 106–116. 10.1177/10883576050200020101.

Grandin, T., & Panek, R. (2013). *The autistic brain.* New York, NY: Houghton Mifflin Harcourt.

Hilton, L. C., Harper, D. J., Kueker, H. R., Lang., R. A., Abbachi., M. A., Todorov, A., & La Vesser, D. P. (2010). Sensory responsiveness as a predictor of social severity in children with high functioning autism spectrum disorders. *Journal of Autism Development Disorder, 40*(8), 937–945. 10.1007/s10803-010-0944-8.

Hirstein, W., Iversen, P., & Ramachandran, S. V. (2001). Autonomic responses of autistic children to people and objects. *Biological Sciences, 268*(1479), 1883–1888.

Hughes, A. D. (2004). *Facilitating developmental attachment. The road to emotional recovery and behavioral change in foster and adopted children.* New York, NY: A Jason Aranson Book.

Klin, A., Lin, D.J., Gorrindo, P., Ramsay, G., & Jones, W. (2009). Two-year-olds with autism orient to non-social contingencies rather than biological motion. *Nature, 459*(7244), 257–261. Retrieved from: http://search.proquest.com/docview/204539039?accountid=12691.

Leekman, R. S., Nieto, C., Libby, J.S., Wing, L., & Gould, J. (2007). Describing the sensory abnormalities of children and adults with autism. *Journal of Autism Development Disorder, 37*(5), 894–910. 10.1007/s10803-006-0218-7.

Marco, J. E., Hinkley, N. B. L., Hill, S. S., & Nagarajan, S. S. (2011). Sensory processing in autism: A review of neurophysiological findings. *Pediatric Research*, 69(5), 48–54.

Miller, J. L., Anzalone, E. M., Lane, J. S., Cermak, A. S., & Osten, T. E. (2007). Concept evolution in sensory integration: A proposed nosology for diagnosis. *The American Journal of Occupational Therapy*, 61(2), 135–140.

Naber, F. B. A., Swinkels, S. H. N., Buitelaar, J. K., Bakermans-Kranenburg, M., van IJzendoorn, M. H., Dietz, C., & van Engeland, H. (2007). Attachment in toddlers with autism and other developmental disorders. *Journal of Autism and Developmental Disorders*, 37(6), 1123–1138. 10.1007/s10803-006-0255-2.

Nadig, A. S., Ozonoff, S., Young, G.S., Rozga, A., Sigman, M., & Rogers, S. J. (2007). A prospective study of response to name in infants at risk for autism. *Archives of Pediatrics and Adolescent Medicine*, 161(4), 378–383. 10.1001/archpedi.161.4.378.

Presmanes, A. G., Walden, T. A., Stone, W. L., & Yoder, P. J. (2007). Effects of different attentional cues on responding to joint attention in younger siblings of children with autism spectrum disorders. *Journal of Autism and Developmental Disorders*, 37(1), 133–144. 10.1007/s10803-006-0338-0.

Robledo, J., Donnellan, M. A., & Strand-Conroy, K. (2012). An exploration of sensory and movement differences from the perspective of individuals with autism. *Frontiers in Integrative Neuroscience*, 6(107), 1–13. 10.3389/fnint.2012.00107.

Rogers, S. J., Ozonoff, S., & Maslin-Cole, C. (1991). A comparative study of attachment behavior in young children with autism or other psychiatric disorders. *Journal of the American Academy of Child and Adolescent Psychiatry*, 26(1), 483–488.

Rogers, J. S., Ozonoff, S., & Maslin-Cole, C. (1993). Developmental aspects of attachment behavior in young children with pervasive developmental disorders. *Journal of the American Academy of Child and Adolescent Psychiatry*, 32(6), 1274–1282.

Rothbaum, F., Weisz, J., Pott, M., Miyake, K., & Morelli, G. (2000). Attachment and culture: Security in the United States and Japan. *The American Psychologist Association*, 55(10), 1093–1104. 10.1037//003-066x.55.10.1093.

Rutgers, A. H., Van Ijzendoorn, M. H., Bakermans-Kranenburg, & Swinkles, M. J. (2007). Autism and attachment: The Attachment Q-sort. *Autism*, 11(2), 187–200. 10.1177/1362361307075713.

Sabatos-De Vito, M., Schipul, E.S., Bulluck, C. J., Belger, A., & Baranek, T. G. (2016). Eye tracking reveals impaired attentional disengagement associated with sensory response patterns in children with autism. *Journal of Autism Development Disorder*, 46(4), 1319–1333. 10.1007/s10803-015-2681-5.

Schore, N. A. (2003). Early relational trauma, disorganized attachment, and the development of a predisposition to violence. In Solomon, F.M. & Siegel, J. D. (Eds.), *Healing Attachment, Trauma, Mind, Body and Brain* (pp. 107–167). New York, NY: W.W. Norton & Company.

Shaver, R. P., & Mikulinger, M. (2002). Attachment related psychodynamics. *Attachment and Human Development*, 4, 133–161. 10.100/14616730210154171.

Shore, A. (2014). Art therapy, attachment and the divided brain. *Journal of the American Art Therapy Association*, 31(2), 91–94.

Siegel, J. D. (2003). An interpersonal neurobiology of psychotherapy: The developing mind and the resolution of trauma. In Solomon, F. M. & Siegel, J.D. (Eds.), *Healing*

Attachment, Trauma, Mind, Body and Brain (pp. 1–56). New York, NY: W.W. Norton & Company.

Sivaratnam, S. C., Newman, K. L., Tonge, J. B., & Rinehart, J. N. (2015). Attachment and emotion processing in children with autism spectrum disorders: Neurological, neuroendocrine, and neurocognitive considerations. *Revised Journal of Autism Development Disorders, 2*(2), 222–242. 10.1007/s40489-015-0048-7.

Sroufe, A. L., Carlson, A. E., Levy, K. A., & Egeland, B. (1999). Implications of attachment theory for developmental psychopathology. *Development and Psychopathology, 11*(1), 1–13.

Stern, N. D. (1977). *The first relationship*. Massachusetts, MA: Harvard University Press.

Stern, N. D. (1985). *The interpersonal world of the infant*. New York, NY: Basic Books.

Teague, J. S., Newman, K. L., Tonge, J. B., & Gray, M. K. (2018). Caregiver mental health, parenting practices, and perceptions of child attachment in children with autism spectrum disorder. *Journal of Autism and Developmental Disorders, 48,* 2642–2652. https://doi.org/10.1007/s10803-018-3517-x.

Tomchek, S. D., & Dunn, W. (2007). Sensory processing in children with and without autism: A comparative study using the short sensory profile. *American Journal of Occupational Therapy, 61*(2), 190–200. 10.5014/ajot.61.2.190.

van der Kolk, B. (2014). *The body keeps the score*. New York, NY: Penguin Books.

Van Ijzendoorn, H. M., Vereijken, L. J. M. C., Bakermans-Kranenberg, J. M., & Risken-Walraven, M. J. (2004). Assessing attachmnet security with the Attachmnet Q sort: Meta-analytic evidence fof the validity of the observer AQS. *Child Development, 75*(4), 1118–1213.

Vaughn, B. E., & Waters, E. (1990). Attachment behavior at home and in the laboratory: Q-sort observations and strange situation classifications of one-year-olds. *Child Development, 61*(6), 1965–1973.

Wakefield, A., Murch, J., Anthony, S. H., Linnell, A., Casson, J., Malik., D. M., & walker-Smith, J. A. (1998). Ileal lymphoid nodular hyperplasia, non-specific colitis, and pervasive developmental disorder in children. *Lancet, 351*(9103), 637–641. Retraction published 2010, *Lancet, 375* (9713), p. 445.

Waters, E., & Deane, K. (1985). Defining and assessing individual differences in attachment relationships: Q-methodology and the organization of behavior in infancy and early childhood. In Bretherton, I. & Waters, E. (Eds.), *Growing points of attachment theory and research. Monographs of the Society for Research in Child Development* (Vol. 50; Serial No. 209; pp. 41–65).

Wing, L. (1996). *The autistic spectrum*. London, UK: Constable and Company Ltd.

3   Art Therapy's Scope to Concurrently Address Impaired Attachment and Comorbid SID

I published my first article on doing art therapy with a child with autism in 2014 based on my work with Nathan, the 12-year-old boy with comorbid ASD and cerebral palsy whom I mentioned in chapter 1. In that article, titled "Facilitating attachment in children with autism through art therapy: A case study" (2014), I presented the idea of forming an attachment with children with ASD through relational artmaking and briefly explored the role of art materials for sensory regulation purposes. Subsequently, in my viewpoint article "A case for art therapy as a treatment for autism spectrum disorder" (Durrani, 2019), I postulated that art therapy can concurrently address sensory regulation, psychomotor development, communication and expression in children with autism. I cited current research and examples from case studies that highlight the broad scope of the discipline. I once again emphasised that art therapists, by virtue of their psychodynamic training, are not only experts in relational development and therefore can address attachment issues but also have a distinct advantage of access to art materials that are multisensory and affect inducing in nature. Hence, I proposed art therapy as the ideal intervention to simultaneously address impaired attachment and sensory challenges in children with ASD.

Below, I touch upon three aspects of art therapy that qualify its position as a fitting therapeutic approach for children with autism. In subsequent chapters, these aspects will be explored in much more detail through the themes of S-BRATA; however, they are included here as a preamble to the framework.

The Magic of Art Materials

When I have the urge to create, I go into my studio with a blank mind, trusting that I will be led once I am among art materials. As my eyes scan the boxes of pastels, containers packed with markers, pencils and charcoal sticks, shelves lined with bottles of paints and stacks of clay, I experience a dull excitement in the pit of my stomach. For a bit, I allow myself to sit with the feeling of being tugged before my hands take over, reaching out to the material that is my calling for that day. Once again, my trust in the power of art materials is renewed as I make art to fulfill the need that instigated the urge in the first place.

Art materials are, to the art therapist, food for the soul. They are the lingua franca that transcend barriers of spoken language, age and ability that art therapists employ in service of their clients. Art therapists work with a wide range of materials available in different textures, colors, smells, tactility and malleability. An art therapy room may have materials ranging from different kinds of pencils, paints, crayons, pastels, charcoal and clay to a variety of surfaces like paper, canvas, board and glass, to more nontraditional materials like shaving foam, gak, found objects, colored sand, beads, buttons, stickers, that may be referred to as pre-art. Almost any material that can be touched and modified can be used for creative expression in one way or another.

Art materials can be categorised by their chemical, physical and sensual qualities; form; texture; temperature; malleability; application and durability. These qualities in turn imbue each material with a unique capacity to evoke or inhibit affective responses that influence expression and behavior. An art therapist understands these capacities and may encourage or discourage the use of specific materials depending on the needs of her clients. For example, paint is fluid and hard to control, whereas a pencil is rigid and lends itself to control. Consequently, paint is emotive and may tap into deep-seated emotions, whereas pencil is restrictive and can facilitate lessening of anxiety through repetitive and controlled mark making. Similarly, engaging with shaving foam can induce hyper-arousal in some children whereas pounding, kneading or molding clay may have the opposite effect of grounding them.

Art therapists who are familiar with the sensory profile of the child with autism and cognizant of their hypo- and hypersensitivities can use art materials to induce or reduce sensations, which in turn may alter the affective state of the child. In the ensuing chapter on "Sensory Regulation," I will illustrate the matter in detail using case vignettes. Once the child is calmer and better regulated, he or she would likely be more open to communication and engagement with the environment.

A Preferred Mode of Communication

Children on the spectrum inherently struggle with relationships and verbal and nonverbal communication. Brain imaging studies reveal that most individuals with autism tend to have extraordinary visuospatial ability and find it easier to process concepts as images rather than words (Kana, Keller, Cherkassky, Minshew & Just, 2006; Kunda & Goel, 2011). Temple Grandin, probably the most well-known autism advocate and person with autism, hypothesised in her book *The Autistic Brain* how there may be three kinds of autistic minds: picture thinker, pattern thinker and fact thinker (Grandin & Panek, 2013). It is not surprising, then, that most interventions and educational approaches for children with autism incorporate visual scaffolding such as Picture Exchange Communication System (PECS), pictorial work systems and activity schedules (Waugh & Peskin, 2015). It makes sense, then, that art therapy, which employs imagery as a means of expression and communication, would be a good fit for individuals whose strength lies in relating to images to understand the world and who may have considerable difficulties with verbal communication. As Henley (2018) put it, "For those on different shades of the spectrum, the creative arts became a critical outlet and preferred personal voice, one that is critical for meaningful self-expression and communication with the outer world" (p. 9). The developmental age of the child with autism will determine his or her stage of artistic development. Whereas some children might be able to make representative art and use images symbolically, others may only be at the level of pre-art or sensory artmaking that resembles playing with art materials. Nonetheless, a multisensory mode of intervention encompassing the entire range of the human sensory experience is likely to be more conducive for working with children with autism who may have challenges across multiple sensory domains as compared to interventions that may be more restrictive.

The Relational Aspect

Art therapy at its current stage of evolution can be considered a hybrid of various psychological approaches ranging from psychoanalytic, developmental, humanistic, analytical, cognitive and systemic among others, with artmaking as the primary mode of expression, communication and reflection. No matter what approach or approaches an art therapist may espouse, the therapeutic alliance between therapist and client lies at the core of the intervention. In fact, an art therapy session can be visualised as a triangle with the art therapist, client and artmaking as the three vertices, each complementing the other. I have already explicated the rationale of addressing SID and impaired attachment concurrently in children with autism. Whereas the art therapist's profound knowledge of art materials equips them to aid sensory regulation in children with sensory challenges and ASD, their psychodynamic training enables them to work in an intersubjective context to create a safe, holding space for the child. Adopting an approach embedded in the phenomena of *mirroring* and *attunement,* the art therapist who is familiar with the explicit and implicit nuances of reciprocal communication can build an attachment relationship with the child. Thus, the art therapist, who understands the language of mark making and imagery, the regulatory capacities of art materials and the dynamics of relational development, is uniquely placed to address both sensory issues and impaired attachment in children with autism.

Art Therapy Practice and Theory that Influenced the S-BRATA

My initial work with children on the spectrum was heavily influenced by Evans and Dubowski's (2001) Interactive Art Therapy Model and Martin's (2009) clinical knowledge of the needs and challenges of children with autism. The relational aspect of the aforementioned authors' works resonated with my personal experience of raising a child with autism. They emphasised the therapist's patient, sensitive and imaginative attitude prioritising the sense of safety for the child with the eventual goal of opening up channels of communication.

Evans and Dubowski's (2001) framework details explicit and implicit nuances of interaction between therapist and child captured through recorded sessions with their clients, which were micro-analysed frame by frame. They emphasised the importance of creating a safe space for the child through an attuned and sensitive approach, paying careful attention to specific details of body position in relation to the child, the child's sensory needs and level of anxiety. They encouraged empowering the child by pre-empting his or her needs and facilitating a holding environment by taking breaks, careful timing and turn taking. Martin (2009), on the other hand, illustrated how to support the artmaking process of the child and facilitate emotional expression and regulation. Particularly valuable are her insights into how sensory modulation may be induced through artmaking and art materials while opening up communication. Martin emphasised the importance of providing "a variety of sensory stimulation in a safe, organised environment using activities that can crack open the door to a child's imagination" (Martin, 2009, p. 20). She suggested experimenting with different art materials to determine their effect on the child, for example, by increasing a child's opportunity to explore materials as a means of facilitating sensory regulation, using art to help process thoughts and feelings and customizing particular art projects that the child expresses interest in to address problems relevant to the child.

Although my stance of tackling sensory issues in children with autism while addressing the attachment relationship echoes Evans and Dubowski's and specifically Martin's approach, the authors do not provide a clear framework in this context for doing art therapy with children on the spectrum. Furthermore, they do not explicitly position the art therapist as an attachment figure, which is a fundamental premise of S-BRATA with major implications for ameliorating an impaired attachment pattern.

Bragge and Fenner's (2009) conceptualised the "Interactive Square," which consists of a quadrangular relationship between the child, the art therapist, the client and the therapist's artwork that reiterates the intersubjective nature of art therapy and resonates with the relational elements of the S-BRATA. They expounded the benefits of co-creative artmaking between child and therapist that in their opinion provides alternative modes of communication between the four elements that constitute the square, not restricting the child to any one specific channel of interaction. This aspect of co-creation and joint artmaking creates opportunities between therapist and child to form a relationship through reciprocal behaviors that are rooted in attachment behaviors. Hence, S-BRATA builds on and extends the work of art therapists who have done wonderful work with children on the spectrum and continue to carry the research forward.

In addition to the insight that I developed from art therapists working within the context of ASD, I would like to acknowledge the role of the

Expressive Therapies Continuum (ETC) (Lusebrink, 2016) in furthering my understanding of my subjects' artwork within the context of their sensory and developmental needs. Following is a summary of the ETC as conceptualised by Lusebrink and Kagan (now Graves Alcorn) in 1978.

Expressive Therapies Continuum

The ETC evolved out of diverse art therapy approaches such as gestalt, psychodynamic, phenomenological and cognitive art therapy (Lusebrink, 2016). Lusebrink, Martinsone, and Dzilna-Silova (2013) credit the art therapy approaches of pioneers such as Florence Cane, Margaret Naumburg, Edith Kramer and Elinor Ulman, among others, that have influenced the operational framework of the ETC. Over a period of 30 years, Lusebrink developed the concept further and systematised the multilevel nature of art expression into a sequential model that parallels the processing of sensory, visual and cognitive information in the brain.

The ETC (Figure 3.1) conceptualises imagery as a psychophysiological phenomenon consisting of three groupings based on the increasing level of cognitive and emotional activity (Lusebrink & Hinz, 2016). The three horizontal levels are classified as kinesthetic/sensory (K/S) level, perceptual/affective (P/A) and cognitive/symbolic (C/Sy) and are spanned vertically by the creative level (CR), which is a synthesis of the different levels of the ETC (Lusebrink, 1992).

Essentially, an artist interacts with art materials at different levels of the Expressive Therapies Continuum. These levels consist of two polarities such

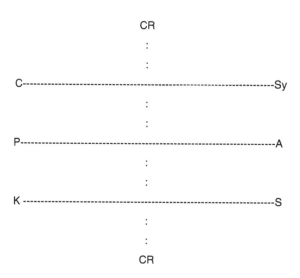

Figure 3.1 The Expressive Therapies Continuum

as the (K/S) that lie at the lowest level of the ETC. These polarities may reinforce or minify each other and exist in relationship with each other as well as the different levels of the ETC (Lusebrink, 1992).

Each level of the ETC contains an emergent function and a healing component. According to Lusebrink (1992), "The healing dimension is specific to a particular level and component of the level; it denotes an optimum intrapersonal functioning on the particular level. The emergent function develops characteristics of the next higher level" (p. 395).

In the context of working with children on the spectrum, the ETC can lend invaluable insights into the developmental stage and needs of the child. For instance, careful observation of the child's interaction with art materials and mark making can inform the therapist of the various levels of the ETC on which the child may be functioning and guide the therapist's intervention accordingly. For instance, those children who tend to remain at the kinesthetic and sensory levels of art making may be doing so to satisfy their sensory needs or, conversely, may not be ready to move up to the perceptual or symbolic levels of the framework due to developmental delays. Thus, knowledge of the ETC can be useful as an ongoing assessment for the therapist throughout the span of the intervention.

Intersubjectivity

The theory of intersubjectivity derives from the progression of psychoanalysis over time as elaborated within object relations and phenomenological frameworks that shifted focus from the primacy of drives to the affective state of individuals (Kenny, 2014). Though it is not within the scope of this book to present any detailed account of the history and development of psychoanalysis, it is important to contextualise intersubjectivity within the evolution of psychodynamic theories for a clearer understanding of how it has influenced the underlying themes of the S-BRATA and its focus on attachment.

Beginning with Sigmund Freud, who is widely considered to be the father of psychoanalysis, modern psychology can be broadly divided into different theoretical approaches that shaped it into its current form. Since Freud, various psychoanalysts and psychologists have proposed disparate and sometimes analogous models of personality development, either emphasising the inner workings of the mind or the environment of the individual or both (Buckley, 1986). Consequently, psychoanalytic practice as it stands today and the ensuing interrelational or intersubjective approaches are the outcome of the instrumental work of some of these experts.

Freud's drive theory was primarily concerned with understanding the origins of psychopathology through the examination of instinctual urges, conflicts and defense mechanisms embedded in the unconscious (Freud, 1940). He was the first person to give the world a schema of personality through his three-tiered conception of the id, ego and super ego that continues to underpin current psychoanalytic thought. Though Freud's theories of psychosexual stages of development were equally revolutionary and con-troversial, he instigated a movement that opened the door for others to delve into the inner workings of the human psyche. Following Freud, psychologists such as Anna Freud, Melanie Klein, Margaret Mahler and Heinz Kohut, among others, developed distinct psychoanalytic theories under the umbrella of *object relations* that advanced psychoanalytic research into the middle of the 20th century.

Whereas Klein was concerned with the interpsychic aspects of the child's relationships with the objects, Mahler, Kohut and Fairbairn theorised upon the role of early object relations within an interpersonal context (Ainsworth, 1969; Kenny, 2014). They began to take psychoanalytic thought outside the individual's or subject's mind into his or her environment that consisted of people or objects around them. In fact, Kohut's theory of *self psychology* was especially instrumental in bringing attention to the centrality of relation-ships, and he underscored that empathy was essential to the healthy devel-opment of personality (Buckley, 1986; Kohut, 1971).

Among the object relationists who put an emphasis on the relational en-vironment of the child's development was an influential English pediatrician and psychoanalyst by the name of D.W. Winnicot introduced the concept of the *holding environment* or the significance of cognizant parenting, wherein he stated "From birth, therefore, the human being is concerned with the problem of the relationship between what is objectively perceived and what is sub-jectively conceived of, and in the solution of this problem there is no health for the human being who has not been started off well enough by a mother" (p. 11). Winnicot's concept of the *good-enough* mother was groundbreaking in that it brought explicit attention to the role of the mother-child relationship and its implications for the healthy development of the child – so much so that for Winnicot, there was no such thing as a baby, only a mother-child unit. Winnicot greatly influenced John Bowlby, the founder of the attachment theory that I have discussed before in some detail.

The term *intersubjective* was first used by Stolorow and Atwood (1992), who belonged to the group of relational thinkers who were greatly influenced by the work of Kohut. One such individual was Harry Stack Sullivan who belonged to the "so-called Interpersonal School of the 1940s and 1950s" (Fonagy & Target, 2003, p. 204). The interpersonalists' major contribution to psychoanalytic practice was the inclusion of the psychoanalyst as a partner rather than an observer in the therapeutic journey of the client (Fonagy & Target, 2003). Once again there was a shift from the intrapsychic to the interpersonal aspects of an individual's psycho-emotional development in which psychotherapy became a relational activity rather than confined to the inner workings of the client's mind. In fact, Stolrow and Atwood (1992) disparaged the concept of "an iso-lated individual mind" (p. 1) and emphasised that psychological phenomena can only be understood within the context of relationships. Intersubjectivity con-tinues to present the modern face of psychoanalysis furthered by the likes of Benjamin (1995) and Mitchell (1988), among others.

What Intersubjective Theorists Say

According to intersubjective theory, a person has a sense of existence because his or her existence is recognised by a *subject* (Stolorow, 2007). To put it simply, an individual exists in relationship to another and in order to thrive must be validated and acknowledged by this other individual (Benjamin, 1988, pp. 19–20). This overarching proposition affirms Bowlby's attachment theory in that the infant's primary relationship constructs meaning via the critical importance of the mother-child relationship, both subjects in their own right. A psychobiologically attuned mother creates a subjective, secure environment for her child to discover his or her sense of self and the selves of the surrounding world (Winnicott, 1971). When a child cries due to hunger or pain, the parent responds to the child's communication by feeding or cuddling the latter, who calms down due to his or her needs being met. Over time, this pattern of reciprocity or *attunement* enables the child to internalise a sense of security that he is not alone and will be looked after. This feeling of safety instills in the child the ability to self-soothe and self-regulate.

The concept of attunement or empathic response runs through Kohut's theory of self psychology, Winnicot's concept of the good enough mother and Bowlby's attachment theory. Benjamin (1988) called it a subliminal act of merging with the other on a psycho-emotional level even as validating each other's existence or sense of being (Benjamin, 1988). Central to the concept of intersubjectivity are the phenomena of mirroring and attunement, which unfold consciously and unconsciously between subjects (Craig, 2009; Gallese, 2009). In fact, both concepts are based on processes of mutual regulation, affective responsivity, empathic resonance, validation and acceptance and are threaded through the theories of attachment and intersubjectivity.

Attunement

Attunement is the cornerstone of the attachment relationship. Stern (1985) described attunement as a continuous process of the mother reflecting the feeling states of the child through identification and response to the latter's inner experiences. A commonplace example of attunement personified is a mother watching her child as he or she attempts to take his or her first steps. The mother responds physically with gestures and actions accompanied by "oohs" and "aahs" to reflect the state of wonderment and fear that the child may be experiencing in attempting to walk. Through her instinctive responses, the mother mirrors back to the baby how he or she may be feeling, sharing his or her inner state (Wright, 2009). Yet another example of attunement is the "let down" reflex that a nursing mother experiences when her breast fills up with milk upon hearing her infant's cry. The more often the mother nurses, the more this reflex attunes to the baby's hunger drive, so much so that the breast fills up with milk in precise relation to the hunger drive of the child. The kind of connection between mother and child, where implicit and explicit communication leads to an in-stinctive response from the other, is the embodiment of an attuned re-lationship (Schore, 2003).

Expressive arts therapist Kossak (2009) described his clinical understanding of attunement as a "felt embodied experience" that includes "a psychological, emotional, and somatic state of consciousness" (p. 14). Observing attunement as it appears in the therapeutic context, Erskine (1998) described a "kinaes-thetic and emotional sensing of others – knowing their rhythm, affect and experience by metaphorically being in their skin" (p. 236). What this means with regards to the therapist-child dyad, then, is the emulation of a mother-child relationship where the therapist is positioned as an attachment figure for the child (Durrani, 2019). An attuned therapist is one who is able to connect at a visceral level with her client within the safety of the therapeutic relationship.

Mirroring

The phenomenon of mirroring is entwined with that of attunement; in fact, it is an aspect of the latter that was empirically affirmed by the discovery of mirror neurons in the human brain. In the 1980s and 1990s, Italian scientists discovered specialised cells in the brains of monkeys that lend credence to the theory that when the monkey picked up a peanut, its same neural pathways were activated as when the monkey saw the researcher pick up the peanut, pointing to the existence of a biological mechanism called the mirror neuron system (MNS) that enabled sharing of the other's feelings or state of affect (Gallese, 2009). The initial experiment conducted by Gallese and his peers at the University of Parma (Gallese, Fadiga, Fogassi, & Rizzolatti, 1996) was later supplanted by the work of Umiltà et al. (2001), who found a subset of mirror neurons that not only discharge in response to a visual stimulus or an action but also to partially hidden actions based on the intention of the subject performing the act. For instance, if you see a person lifting an ice cream cone to his mouth but he turns away so that you do not actually see him licking it, you may still begin to salivate, anticipating the completion of the individual's goal of eating the ice cream.

This interpersonal link between a perceived action and the understanding of the intention and goal behind that action is what Gallese called *embodied simulation*, which stems from the MNS (Gallese, 2005). As an example, embodied simulation mechanisms in the mirror neuron system enable a person to perceive the other person's raised hand, say, as the "high five" it is intended to be rather than an act of aggression. The feeling of happiness that initiated the high five in the subject who started the act would be shared with the receiver of the act. Gallese (2009) elaborated:

> Thus, we have a neurally instantiated we-centric space. I posit that
> a common underlying functional mechanism – embodied simulation –

mediates our capacity to share the meaning of actions, intentions, feelings, and emotions with others, identification, empathy, and "we-ness" are the basic ground of our development and being. (p. 520)

This "we-ness," as Gallese called it, is the act of merging of boundaries between subject and object in an empathically attuned relationship in which the state of one can be experienced by the other not just mentally but physically as well (Gallese, 2012).

With regards to children with autism, one may wonder whether the difficulty they have with reading facial expressions and emotions of other people has something to do with an impaired MNS. Gallese (2006) posited that children on the spectrum might have embodied simulation deficits that make it difficult for them to simulate other people's actions and intentions suggesting a faulty MNS. Oberman, Pineda, and Ramachandaran (2007) reaffirmed Gallese's contention by citing five studies that claim a dysfunction of the MNS in individuals with ASD.

The MNS is made up of neurons that respond individually or collectively to visual, auditory and somatosensory stimuli (Gallese, 2005). For instance, some neurons may be activated with the movement of three-dimensional objects, whereas others might respond to touch or tactile stimulation (Gallese, 2005; Warren et al., 2006). Kohler et al. (2002) discovered that another set of mirror neurons, the audio-visual mirror neurons, activate upon hearing a sound associated with a particular action. For example, the sound of an electric drill in an adjacent room may give rise to an image of someone drilling a hole in the wall even though the act is not visible to the listener.

Interestingly, a study by Warren et al. (2006) explored the domain of auditory-motor mirror neurons that respond to the observation of an action and hearing the sound of the same action. Their functional magnetic resonance imaging study demonstrated that the auditory-motor mirror neurons are activated in response to positive vocalisations that also mediate appropriate orofacial gestures. For example, in most cases, listening to cheering or laughter will invoke a laugh or a smile just like an applause or expressions of commendation.

The findings of Warren et al. (2006) provide evidence of a mirroring system that responds to the positive emotional states of others and could provide a mechanism for the formation of empathy and social bonds between individuals. The knowledge that positive experiences may enhance the function of the MNS is encouraging for children on the spectrum whose MNS has been implicated for their difficulty in reciprocal relationships and reading the minds of others. Hence, art therapists can focus on creating affirmative relational experiences in the session to facilitate the function of the MNS. Attunement and mirroring go hand in hand in creating an intersubjective experience for the child and therapist that is optimal for the development of an attachment relationship.

Conclusion

Art therapy research and practice elucidates the positive effects of an art therapy intervention on the cognitive, behavioral, and psychological development of the child with autism. Art therapy is an ideal approach for children with autism due to its multisensory nature. It caters to the needs of individuals who are likely more comfortable with a nonverbal approach and can derive benefit from the regulatory qualities of art materials as well as the relational aspect of art therapy practice. The S-BRATA draws from the work of art therapists who emphasise the sensory and regulatory aspects of art materials and artmaking within an intersubjective context in which the therapist creates a safe holding environment for the child to express and communicate freely. The therapist can emulate a mother-child relationship by mirroring and attuning to the child formulating an attachment relationship that emanates from embodied intelligence and empathic resonance.

References

Ainsworth, M. S. (1969). Object relations, dependency, and attachment: Atheoretical review of the infant-mother relationship. *Child Development, 40,* 969–1025.

Benjamin, J. (1988). *The bonds of love.* New York, NY: Pantheon Books.

Benjamin, J. (1995). Recognition and destruction: An outline of intersubjectivity. *In like subjects, love objects: Essays on recognition and sexual difference* (pp. 27–48). New Haven, CT: Yale University Press.

Betts, D., Harmer, R., & Schumelevich, G. (2014). The contributions of art therapy in treatment, assessment, and research with people who have autism spectrum disorders. In Hu, V. W. (Ed.), *Frontiers in autism research: New horizons for diagnosis and treatment* (pp. 627–655). Hackensack, NJ: World Scientific.

Bragge, A., & Fenner, P. (2009). The emergence of the 'interactive square' as an approach to art therapy with children on the autistic spectrum. *International Journal of Art Therapy, 14*(1), 17–28. 10.1080/17454830903006323.

Buckley, P. (1986). *Essential papers on object relations.* New York, NY: New York University Press.

Craig, M. G. (2009). Intersubjectivity, phenomenology and multiple disabilities. *International Journal of Art Therapy, 14,* 64–73. doi: 10.1080/17454830903329204.

Durrani, H. (2014). Facilitating attachment in children with autism through art therapy: A case study. *Journal of Psychotherapy Integration, 24*(2), 99. 10.1037/a0036974.

Durrani, H. (2019). A case for art therapy as a treatment for autism spectrum disorder, *Art Therapy.* doi: 10.1080/07421656.2019.1609326.

Erskine, R. (1998). Attunement and involvement: Therapeutic responses to relational needs. *International Journal of Psychotherapy, 3*(3), 235–244.

Evans, K., & Dubowski, J. (2001). *Art therapy with children on the autisticspectrum.* London, UK: Jessica Kingsley.

Fonagy, P., & Target, M. (2003). *Psychoanalytic theories. Perspectives from developmental psychopathology.* London: Whurr Publishers.

Freud, S. (1940). *An outline in psychoanalysis*. New York, NY: Norton.

Gallese, V. (2005). Embodied simulation: From neurons to phenomenal experience. *Phenomenology and Cognitive Sciences*, 4(1), 23–48. 10.1007/s11097-005-4737-z.

Gallese, V., Fadiga, L., Fogassi, L., & Rizzolatti, G. (1996). Action recognition in the premotor cortex. *Brain*, *119*, 593–609. doi: 10.1093/brain/119.2.593.

Gallese, V. (2006). Intentional attunement: A neurophysiological perspective on social cognition and its disruption in autism. *Brain Research*, *1079*(1), 15–24. 10.1016/j.brainres.2006.01.054.

Gallese, V. (2009). Mirror neurons, embodied simulation and the neural basis of social identity. *Psychoanalytic Dialogues*, *19*(5), 519–536, 2009. 10.1080/10481880903231910

Gallese, V. (2012). Embodied simulation theory and intersubjectivity. *Reti, Saperi, Linguaggi*, 4(2), 57–64.

Grandin, T., & Panek, R. (2013). *The autistic brain*. New York, NY: Houghton Mifflin Harcourt.

Hass-Cohen, N., & Findlay, C. J. (2015). *Art therapy and the neuroscience of relationships, creativity and resiliency*. New York, NY: W. W. Norton & Company, Inc.

Henley, R. D. (2018). *Creative response activities for children on the spectrum*. New York, NY: Routledge.

Kana, R. K., Keller, T. A., Cherkassky, V. L., Minshew, N. J., & Just, M. A. (2006). Sentence comprehension in autism: Thinking in pictures with decreased functional connectivity. *Brain*, *129*, 2484–2493. 10.1093/brain/awl164.

Kenny, T. D. (2014). *From id to intersubjectivity. Talking about the talking cure with master clinicians*. London: Karnac Books Ltd.

Kohler, E., Keysers, C., Umiltà, M. A., Fogassi, L., Gallese, V., & Rizzolatti, G. (2002). Hearing sounds, understanding actions: Action representation in mirror neurons. *Science*, *297*(5582), 846–848. 10.1126/science.1070311.

Kohut, H. (1971). *The analysis of the self*. Chicago, IL: University of Chicago Press.

Kossak, S. M. (2009). Therapeutic attunement: A transpersonal view of expressive arts therapy. *The Arts in Psychotherapy*, *36*, 13–18. 10.1016/j.aip.2008.09.003.

Kuo, N., & Plavnick, J. B. (2015). Using an antecedent art intervention to improve the behavior of a child with autism. *Art Therapy: Journal of the American Art Therapy Association*, *32*(2), 13–19. 10.1080/07421656.2015.1028312.

Kunda, M., & Goel, A. K. (2011). Thinking in pictures as a cognitive account of autism. *Journal of Autism and Developmental Disorders*, *41*, 1157–1177. 10.1007/s10803-010-1137-1.

Lusebrink, V. B. (2016). Expressive therapies continuum. In Gussak, E. D. & Rosal, L. M. (Eds.), *The Wiley handbook of art therapy* (pp. 57–67). UK: Wiley- Blackwell.

Lusebrink, B. V. & Hinz, D. L. (2016). The expressive therapies continuum as a framework in the treatment of trauma. In King, L. J. (Ed.) *Art therapy, trauma, and neuroscience* (pp. 42–66). New York, NY: Routledge.

Lusebrink, V. B. (1992). A systems oriented approach to the expressive therapies: The expressive therapies continuum. *The Arts in Psychotherapy*, *18*(5), 395–403. doi: 10.1016/0197-4556(91)90051-b.

Lusebrink, V., Martinsone, K., & Dzilna-Silova, I. (2013). The expressive therapies continuum (ETC): Interdisciplinary basis of ETC. *International Journal of Art Therapy*, *182*(2), 75–85. 10.1080/17454832.2012.713370.

Martin, N. (2009). *Art as an early intervention tool for children with autism*. London, UK: Jessica Kingsley.

Mitchell, A. S. (1988). *Relational concepts in psychoanalysis: An integration*. Cambridge, MA: Harvard University Press.

Oberman, M. l., Pineda, A. J., & Ramachandaran, S. V. (2007). The human mirror neuron system: A link between action observation and social skills. *Social Cognitive and Affective Neuroscience, 2*(1), 62–66. 10.1093/scan/ns1022.

Schore, N. A. (2003). Early relational trauma, disorganized attachment, and the development of a predisposition to violence. In Solomon, F. M. & Siegel, J. D. (Eds.), *Healing attachment, trauma, mind, body and brain* (pp. 107–167). New York, NY: W.W. Norton & Company.

Schweizer, C., Knorth, E. J., & Spreen, M. (2014). Art therapy with children with autism spectrum disorders: A review of clinical case descriptions on 'what works'. *The Arts in Psychotherapy, 41*(5), 577–593. 10.1016/j.aip.2014.10.009.

Stern, N. D. (1985). *The interpersonal world of the infant*. New York, NY: Basic Books.

Stolrow, D. R. (2007). *Trauma and human existence*. New York, NY: Routledge.

Stolrow, D. R., & Atwood, G. (1992). *Contexts of being: The intersubjective foundations of psychological life*. Hills-dale, NJ: Analytic Press.

Umiltà, M. A., Kohler, E., Gallese, V., Fogassi, L., Fadiga, L., Keysers, C., et al. (2001). "I know what you are doing": A neurophysiological study. *Neuron, 32*(1), 91–101. 10.1016/S0896-6273(01)00337-3.

Warren, E. J., Sauter, A. D., Eisner, F., Wiland, J., Dresner, A. M., Wise, S. R., et al. (2006). Positive emotions preferentially engage an auditory-motor "mirror" system. *Journal of Neuroscience, 26*(50), 13067–13075. 10.1523/JNEUROSCI.3907-06.2006

Waugh, C., & Peskin, J. (2015). Improving the social skills of children with HFASD: An intervention study. *Journal of Autism Development Disorder, 45*, 2961–2980. 10.1007/s10803-015-2459-9.

Winnicot, D. W. (1971). *Playing and reality*. Tavistock Publications Ltd.

Winnicot, D. W. (2005). *Playing and reality*. Oxford, UK: Routledge Classics.

Wright, K. (2009). *Mirroring and attunement. Self-realization in psychoanalysis and art*. New York, NY: Routledge.

4 Methodology and Procedures

The S-BRATA evolved from research that was based on three case studies of Teo, Raj and Alex. All three boys were chosen through purposive or judgmental sampling that is used for unique and specialised populations "to gain a deeper understanding and not to generalize the findings" (Ishak & Abu Bakar, 2014, p. 32). I used closed groups on Facebook to connect with caregivers of children with autism wherein I specified the requirements for eligibility for my research: a diagnosis of ASD and the presence of considerable comorbid SID. The specified age group of children was 3–8 years. Interested caregivers were asked to come for a preliminary interview and bring along their child for an informal observation.

Teo, Raj and Alex's levels of SID were determined through the preliminary interview with their caregiver and by observation in the first meeting. "It was assumed that a child with considerable sensory regulation issues would have impaired attachment. As such the attachment was not measured through formalised testing due to lack of resources" (Durrani, 2019). All three boys fit the profile that I was looking for and were chosen to be my research subjects. Initially, another boy, Sean, was also inducted in the study but sessions with him had to be discontinued due to familial issues that prevented him from regular commitment. All research subjects were confirmed not to have received any art therapy intervention prior to the study.

Setting

The setting for conducting the sessions was my art therapy studio where I see my private clients. The studio consists of a small waiting room and a spacious therapy room big enough to accommodate two sets of tables and chairs (one for adults and one for children) for artmaking, a couple of armchairs and bean bags, leaving a large space in the middle that allows for artmaking and playing on the floor. The floor itself is covered with soft rubber matting, similar to what one would find in a yoga studio, and a third of the walls are lined with floor to ceiling mirrors that can be incorporated in sensory play and artmaking. It is the kind of space that is large enough to play catch yet cosy enough to chill out on a bean bag.

Art Therapy Materials

The studio is equipped with a large variety of art materials, ranging from typical art supplies to novel materials that can be incorporated into sensory activities such as goop/slime, colored sand, shaving foam, pastas and lentils for sticking and pasting, beads, buttons and so on. There are some musical instruments and play therapy toys on display that clients are free to use during the session. Most of the art material is displayed and easily accessible other than the materials that may be fragile or can cause harm to certain clients. Art materials are restocked regularly and additional materials brought in as required.

Data Collection Procedure

The research that informed the S-BRATA was based on 12 sessions with Teo, Raj and Alex, each session approximating 45 minutes, once a week. As mentioned earlier, sessions with Sean had to be terminated prematurely due to irregular attendance that invalidated the efficacy of the intervention, and his case was removed from the study. Data was collected through the following:

a) Pre- and post-therapy interviews with caregivers. The pre-therapy interviews consisted of informal conversations about the child's history, developmental and psychosocial behaviors, with special attention given to the child's sensory profile. Caregivers were given a clear description of the intervention, its purpose, the process, possible risks involved and rights of the subject, which were clearly delineated and explicitly stated in the consent form. The post-therapy interview was conducted to collect feedback from the caregivers about changes in the child's psycho-emotional, developmental or sensory related behaviors.
b) Video recordings of the 12 sessions were made using an i-Phone 5 mounted on a tripod. Fortunately, the mirror-lined walls of the studio proved to be a huge asset since tactful placement of the tripod allowed for capturing most of the activity within the room through the mirrors. An aggregate video of 12 sessions with each child was made after the conclusion of the study and shared with the caregiver as well as another art therapist to confirm accuracy of my claims with the clinical notes.
c) Artwork of the subjects was digitally recorded and kept safely before return to their caregivers.
d) Detailed clinical notes were made after each session and shared with the art therapist together with the aggregate videos. The videos and clinical notes were reviewed concurrently multiple times during the data analysis.

Case Study

A case study is a detailed exploration of a research problem that is analyzed through a comprehensive collection of data that may consist of interviews, observations, clinical notes, texts, artwork, referral documents, letters and other relevant information that may add value to understanding the phenomena (Gilroy, 2006; Kapitan, 2014). Kapitan (2014) enumerated three types of case studies: intrinsic case study, in which a case is pre-selected to study a specific issue; instrumental case study, in which the aim of the researcher is to gain a deeper understanding of an issue and participatory case research, in which the participant also acts as the co-researcher with firsthand experience of a particular situation. Case studies may be retrospective in nature, where the researcher's goal is to re-examine past events, or ongoing, where the participant may contribute to the analysis of the researcher. Moreover, case studies may be single-case or multi-case; in either case, it is critical for the researcher to clearly define the problem to be studied in order to understand the phenomena particularly rather than generally (Stake, 1995).

I chose multi-case study as a method for collecting data for my research problem because it lends itself to an intensive observation and qualitative analysis. The methodology allowed me to explore and document in detail my engagement with Teo, Raj and Alex that I subsequently analyzed through grounded theory methodology.

Grounded Theory Methodology

I used grounded theory methodology to generalise the data from the case studies through comparison and analytical generalisation (see Figure 4.1) (Ishak & Abu Bakar, 2014; Yin, 2009). Grounded theory is a qualitative method of research that uses rigorous analysis of empirical data through systematic data collection and lateral analysis that informs the process of research. According to Corbin and Strauss (1990), grounded theory should be able to explain social phenomena through detailed theoretical explanation. The researcher has to keep in mind that the phenomena can undergo change with evolving situations as it is not static; therefore, strict determinism is not possible in grounded theory methodology. The authors stated, "A grounded theory should explain as well as describe. It may also implicitly give some degree of predictability, but only with regard to specific conditions" (Corbin & Strauss, 1990, p. 5).

Data can be collected through interviews, videos, books, observations, newspaper or any other source that informs the research question. Each concept that is discovered in the process of research is documented and incorporated into the theory under labels, categories and groups that are integrated into the theory in the light of analytic narratives.

Data Analysis

Thirty-six analytic tables based on the 36 sessions with Teo Raj and Alex were created to code the data from the videos and the clinical notes into

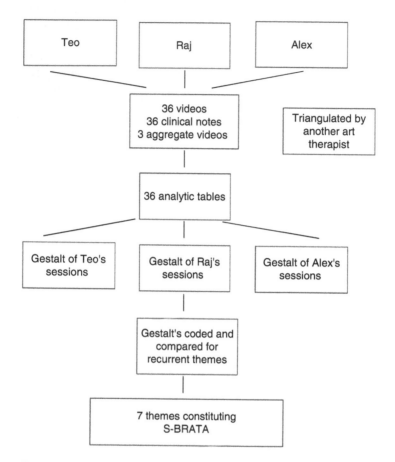

Figure 4.1   Illustration of grounded theory methodology including data collection and data analysis procedure (Durrani, 2019)

analysable categories (see Table 4.1). The categories in the tables were informed from the topics in the attachment Q-Sort questionnaire, which is used to measure the attachment patterns in children on the spectrum (Vaughn & Waters, 1990). Next, three gestalt tables were created based on the key concepts that arose from the 36 analytic tables (see Table 4.2). The data from the gestalts were coded and compared for recurrence and relevance and resulted in the generation of the seven themes of the S-BRATA, namely, (a) sense of safety, (b) the child's sensory profile, (c) art materials as entry point for engagement, (d) mirroring and attunement, (e) flexibility, (f) structure and boundaries and (g) art product not a focus.

Below are the gestalts of Teo, Raj and Alex's sessions. They were created to broadly encapsulate my experience with the boys through the 12 therapy sessions to generate key points that were compared and coded to identify the

Was the child resistant to enter the room?	(a) No
	(b) Is comfortable with unfamiliar environment
	(c) Felt safe
Was the child comfortable with proximity to the therapist?	(a) Approached me when I offered material and once when he seemed to ask for a hug at the end of the session
	(b) Art material provided motivation for proximity
	(c) Art material as entry point to engagement
Did the therapist mirror the child's vocalisations actions, emotions?	(a) Yes
	(b) Tried to attune by mimicking R's vocalisations but felt out of synch
	(c) R not responsive to my attempts
Did child respond to directives?	(a) Came to me when I called his name and directed attention to the art material
	(b) Wouldn't call it a response to directives
	(c) Not motivated to interact with me
Did child respond to turn taking?	(a) No
	(b) Did not seem interested in reciprocity
	(c) Not motivated/dysregulated
Did the child imitate the therapist?	(a) No
	(b) Did not seem interested in reciprocity
	(c) Not motivated/dysregulated
Did the therapist use things other than art material such as musical instruments and games, toys?	(a) Yes, I used the drum
	(b) Not necessary to restrict to art materials
	(c) Flexibility in approach is necessary
Was there an attempt at joint attention from child?	(a) No
	(b) Is not motivated to engage with me
	(c) May be skill not developed yet
Did the child display anger/crying/tantrums?	(a) No
	(b) Is ok with unfamiliar surroundings
	(c) Felt safe
Was engagement with the art material only at a sensory level?	(a) Yes
	(a) Sensory quality was the main attraction
	(b) Not interested in mark making
Was there any art product at the end of the session?	(a) No
	(b) Sensory play was focus
	(c) Art product not a goal
Comments	I was calmer than the first session and reminded myself that it was ok to take things slowly. Doubts about the suitability of the approach for R entered my mind because he seemed so uninterested in my attempts to engage.

Table 4.1 Sample of an analytic table

Gestalt of sessions with Teo	Gestalt of sessions with Raj	Gestalt of sessions with Alex
Teo had to feel safe in the environment in order to engage with the me.	Raj felt safe in the environment in order to engage with the me.	Alex felt safe in the environment in order to engage with the me.
Familiarity with the Teo's sensory profile was necessary for me to understand challenges with communication. I used art materials to induce and modulate affect.	Familiarity with Raj's sensory profile was necessary to understand his highs and lows. I was not able to regulate Raj sufficiently with art materials.	Familiarity with Alex's sensory profile was necessary to manage his regulation. I was able to manage Alex's arousal levels through art materials.
Art materials were an entry point to engagement.	Art materials were an entry point to engagement although were not a significant attraction to get Raj to sustain a relationship with me.	Art materials were an entry point to engagement.
	Raj required more structure than others. Hence, art therapists may have to adjust their approach to suit the specific needs of the child with autism as in Raj's case	Firm boundaries worked for Alex and helped in regulating his affect.
I felt anxious, rejected and frustrated in the session. I was aware of feelings of countertransference.	I had strong countertransference and felt rejected.	I was mindful of my bodily responses and countertransference.
Flexibility in approach was necessary to meet Teo where he was at. If he was not comfortable working on the table then I used the floor, if not the floor then the wall. I did not restrict themselves to art materials only and was open to using toys or musical instruments.	Art therapy may not work for every child with autism. Art materials were not sufficient to address Raj's sensory needs.	Flexibility in approach was required. Some things that worked in one session, did not in the next. Constant adjustments had to be made.
Mirroring Teo's vocalizations and actions helped attune to the latter's inner state. I felt a sense of embodied communication where a subliminal bond was being created in replication of a mother-child relationship.	My bodily rhythm, sensations and affect provided clues to what may be happening in the session and was possibly reflective of Raj's affect as well. I struggled to attune with Raj.	I had to pay attention to Alex's body language to attune to him and adjusted my response accordingly. Rupture and repair are part of the process of attachment.
Art product was not necessary.	Art product was not necessary.	Art product was secondary.

Table 4.2 Comparison table based on the gestalt of the 36 analytic tables

seven themes of the S-BRATA. Vignettes in the ensuing chapters will expound the key points below that underpin the themes of the framework.

Gestalts of Teo's Sessions

Teo was resistant to enter the art therapy room initially possibly because he was not familiar with the environment and did not feel safe. I had to ask his mother to sit in the first few sessions and after that keep the door to the waiting room slightly ajar till he seemed comfortable. During the first half of the 12 sessions, Teo appeared to be oblivious to my presence and was not interested to engage despite my attempts to lure him with art materials. I mimicked his vocalisations and mirrored his movements as he ran around the room seemingly enclosed in his world. I was keenly aware of Teo's sensory needs and the potential in using non-traditional art materials to motivate him. Eventually, pre-art materials like shaving foam and play dough caught Teo's attention and became the entry point for his engagement with me. Shaving foam and play dough provided him the tactile input that he sought. I persevered in my attempts to attune to Teo, incorporating play such as tag and musical instruments and toys to draw him in. Teo was not restricted to any surface such as a particular table or part of the room for artmaking (he used the mirrored lined walls to spread paint and foam). I sensed a very gradual shift in Teo's attention as sessions progressed, at times vacillating between frustration and anxiety at his relative disinterest in me or artmaking. I was mindful of my countertransference toward Teo and reminded myself to be patient and optimistic. Around session five, Teo's mother reported that he had begun to touch his food to feel the texture, which was a new behavior since Teo had never paid attention to it before. It was in this very session that I sensed Teo entered the room willingly and I was able to safely close the door to the waiting room. Session nine was a breakthrough session where Teo started responding to his name and to my directions for the first time. Subsequently, there was an increase in reciprocity, engagement and some joint attention. Towards the end of the sessions, there was an indication of emerging play when Teo threw back a ball at me. Teo's mother was thrilled with his progress at home. She reported that he had begun to imitate children in the park and had asked for water, something that he had never done before.

Key Points

- Teo had to feel safe in the environment in order to engage with me.
- Art materials were an entry point for engagement.
- Teo was motivated to use non-traditional art materials with strong tactile input.
- I did not restrict myself to art material only and was open to using toys and musical instruments.

- Flexibility in approach was necessary and I followed Teo's lead in the sessions. Teo had access to the entire studio for artmaking.
- I mirrored Teo's vocalisations and actions to attune to him attempting to emulate a mother-child relationship.
- At times I felt anxious, rejected and frustrated in the sessions. I was aware of feelings of countertransference and my bodily reactions to events in the sessions.
- Art product was neither the focus nor necessary.

Gestalt of Raj's Sessions

Raj was comfortable to enter the art therapy room from the very beginning of the sessions but did not seem interested in engaging with me. Art materials eventually created the opportunity for proximity with him and engagement but his response felt forced rather than motivated. I had strong countertransference towards him and began to have doubts about the suitability of my approach since Raj continued to be evasive and preoccupied with stimming. I struggled with mirroring his vocalisations and actions possibly because I was overwhelmed with mirroring his anxiety and hyperarousal. By session three, Raj became a bit responsive before things started to fall apart in session five. Raj appeared to be more dysregulated than before and I suspected that I was not able to induce sensory regulation in him through art materials. He seemed to require more movement than I could incorporate in artmaking. I also began to realise that possibly the sessions were not structured enough for him and that he would require firmer boundaries. I was not sure how to implement structure that would work for Raj as he was not easily motivated to engage with me. However, there were some sessions where I felt, despite Raj's relative lack of inclination to make art or indulge in reciprocal behaviors, that he had developed some emotional connection with me particularly when he sought proximity through hugs. Also, in one session when he sat close to me and very calmly listened to a lullabye, I sensed a connection or bonding pervading through the interaction. By the end of Raj's 12 sessions, I was left feeling that although there were occasions pointing to some attuned relational activity between us, they were rare. Perhaps art materials and artmaking, or the way I used them, were not a sufficient draw for Raj to engage with me, or maybe the duration of therapy was not long enough for me to attune to Raj.

Key Points

- Raj felt safe in the sessions and came willingly for therapy.
- Art materials were an entry point for engagement with Raj but were not a significant attraction to sustain an attachment relationship.
- Raj possibly required more structure and boundaries in the sessions than I could provide.

- Art materials or the way I used them were not sufficient to address Raj's sensory needs.
- My bodily rhythm, sensations and affect provided clues into how the sessions were progressing and were possibly reflective of Raj's anxiety levels.
- Art product was not the focus.

Gestalt of Sessions with Alex

Alex came happily for the sessions. His reciprocal skills were well developed; he could listen to directives, do turn taking and had joint attention. However, I could sense his underlying anxiety through the sessions that was reflected in a short attention span, tendency to get bored quickly with one activity and a general state of hyperarousal. Alex enjoyed making art and responded well to the regulatory capacity of art materials. I found myself adjusting my tone of voice to regulate Alex's affect. I consistently mirrored his actions and used exaggerated affect and effusive praise to keep him engaged. I was mindful of my own bodily responses and countertransference toward Alex. In session four, Alex's behavior took a turn when he seemed to want to seek conflict and push boundaries. I noted that Alex struggled with transitions; for instance, there was conflict at entering the room and leaving the room. According to Alex's mother, this was typical of his behavior especially when he became comfortable with someone. The sessions became unpredictable and I had to start imposing firm boundaries to manage Alex's behavior; for example, I cut short a session when he was extremely disruptive and sent him home. I continued to use art materials to regulate Alex's level of arousal. Sessions with Alex seemed to reflect a pattern of rupture and repair in attachment. I induced repair through maintaining boundaries and phasing out transitions that were hard for Alex; for example, I avoided conflict at transitions and began to prepare him much in advance for closure of session. Also, I learned how to distract and divert his attention rather than address his negative behavior directly. Before the last session, Alex's mother reported that he really enjoyed coming for art therapy and that he had been behaving very well the past week. During the duration of the 12 sessions, Alex communicated his fondness for me several times. There were many sessions that he did not want to go home from therapy, which could have been indicative of his difficulty with transitions; however, I do believe that he had developed an attachment to me.

Key Points

- Art materials were an entry point for engagement.
- I had to pay close attention to Alex's tone and body language in order to to attune to him.
- Alex's therapeutic trajectory was unpredictable and I had to learn to be comfortable with that. Rupture and repair are part of the process of attachment.

- Firm boundaries and some structure worked for Alex.
- Flexibility in approach was required. Some things that worked in one session did not in the next, and constant adjustments had to be made.
- Art product was secondary.

Conclusion

The S-BRATA was generated from qualitative research built on Teo, Raj and Alex's art therapy sessions over an approximate period of three months. Grounded theory methodology was used to analyse thick data from the three case studies that consisted of video recordings and clinical notes. The videos and clinical notes were reviewed by another art therapist who confirmed the accuracy of my clinical analysis.

References

Corbin, J., & Strauss, A. (1990). Grounded theory research: Procedures, canons, and evaluative criteria. *Qualitative Sociology, 13*(1), 3–21.

Durrani, H. (2019). Art therapy's scope to address attachment in children with ASD and comorbid SID. *Journal of Art Therapy.* 10.1080/07421656.2019.1677063.

Gilroy, A. (2006). *Art therapy, research and evidence-based practice.* London, UK: Sage Publications.

Ishak, M. N., & Abu Bakar, Y. A. (2014). Developing sampling frame for case study: Challenges and conditions. *World Journal of Education, 4*(3), 293–295. 10.5430/wje. v4n3p29.

Kapitan, L. (2014). *Introduction to art therapy research.* New York, NY: Routledge.

Stake, R. E. (1995). *The art of case study research.* Thousand Oaks, CA: Sage Publications.

Vaughn, B. E., & Waters, E. (1990). Attachment behavior at home and in the laboratory: Q-sort observations and strange situation classifications of one-year-olds. *Child Development, 61*(6), 1965–1973.

Yin, R. K. (2009). *Case study research: Design and methods* (4th ed.). Thousand Oaks, CA: SAGE Publications.

Part II

The Seven Themes of the S-BRATA

5 Sense of Safety

It is important to remember that autism is placed on a spectrum because it manifests in individuals in variations and degrees. Consequently, any intervention that adopts a one-size-fits-all approach is bound to be inadequate and limiting. The same principle applies to the S-BRATA, and therefore it must be emphasised that it is not meant to be prescriptive nor restrictive. All seven themes of the approach arose out of my experience with children on the spectrum, and most likely therapists working with similarly diagnosed children will find some similarities but also many differences from my research subjects: Teo, Raj and Alex. In fact, one of the reasons why S-BRATA is a preliminary framework is because it has room for expansion and development as research continues to advance in the field of art therapy and autism. Therefore, it is meant to be taken as a guideline for working with children with autism, keeping in mind the essence of the themes rather than specifics, considering the variability inherent in the spectrum. All seven themes run concurrent to each other and are not sequential in nature; though I begin with the *sense of safety*, it must pervade throughout the sessions together with *mirroring and attunement* or *flexibility* and so on. Most of the primary themes have been divided into sub-themes to facilitate in-depth analysis and description (see Figure 5.1).

Teo's, Raj's and Alex's cases provided the data for the grounded theory methodology that generated the themes. As I worked through the 12 sessions with each child, I adjusted and adapted my approach, building on my learning from the previous sessions. The missteps that happened were equally important in informing the approach as were the successes. After a brief introduction to Teo, Raj and Alex, I have attempted to provide a reflective account of my experiences through vignettes from their sessions that illustrate the following themes: (a) sense of safety, (b) the child's sensory profile, (c) art materials as entry point for engagement, (d) mirroring and attunement (e) flexibility, (f) structure and boundaries and (g) art product not a focus (see Figure 5.1).

Teo

Teo was 5 years old when I saw him. Slight-framed and frail in appearance, he showed no apparent interest in his environment. Although verbal, Teo did

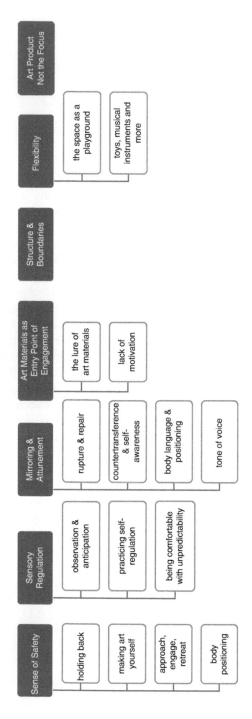

Figure 5.1 The seven themes of the S-BRATA and their sub-themes

not use language functionally; instead, he perseverated on nursery rhymes that he had picked up from school and home. Teo had begun occupational therapy (OT) just prior to coming for art therapy and had had no other interventions since he was diagnosed with ASD at 2 years and 4 months of age. Teo's mother shared that he did not respond to his name, never asked for anything, not even to eat or drink, and did not show any discomfort upon soiling his diaper. Essentially, Teo appeared to be closed off or *shut down* from the outside world. He was highly sensory seeking in that he craved touch and movement indicating that he was probably tactile hyposensitive and had challenges in vestibular and proprioceptive domains. Teo lacked body awareness and would often walk over play dough and wet paint on paper laid on the floor.

Raj

Raj was diagnosed with autism at 3 years 10 months of age and was 7 years old when he came for art therapy. He had been receiving OT for a few years and Relationship Development Intervention (RDI) for 1.5. Raj's mother shared that he had great vestibular and proprioceptive needs. In my pre-therapy interview with his mother where Raj accompanied her, I observed that he preferred to constantly run around the art therapy room while I spoke to her. Raj had limited language as in, he could understand single command instructions, but his verbal ability was limited to mimic words like "yes" and "no."

Alex

At 7 years of age, Alex presented as a strong and robust boy with a jovial disposition. Alex had age-appropriate language skills and his primary challenge was difficulty with self-regulation. Alex's mother shared that he struggled with separation from her in school and was generally not good with transitions. Alex was oral seeking (he ground his teeth excessively) and had significant proprioceptive needs and a short attention span.

Sense of Safety

The sense of safety or the feeling of being protected is an inherent need of the human infant who seeks it from the most readily available source, who in most cases is the primary caregiver. This need for being *held* physically, emotionally and psychologically, translates into a secure attachment pattern when met with the attuned responses of a caregiver. An impairment in this first relationship can result in long term feelings of insecurity and anxiety in infants, with negative consequences for their psychoemotional development that may last into adulthood. For children with autism and comorbid SID, who have a higher likelihood of having an impaired attachment pattern (Durrani, 2019), the sense of safety may be compromised and exacerbated by an incoherent sensory system, difficulty with theory of mind (TOM) and relational and communication difficulties. Self-stories of individuals with autism lend profound insight into the challenges inherent in the spectrum. Naoki Higashida, a teenager with autism, in his memoir *The Reason I Jump* shared:

> One of the biggest misunderstandings you have about us is your belief that our feelings aren't as subtle and complex as yours. Because how we behave can appear so childish in your eyes, you tend to assume that we're childish on the inside, too. But of course, we experience the same emotions that you do. And because people with autism aren't skillful talkers, we may in fact be more sensitive than you are. Stuck here inside these unresponsive bodies of ours, with feelings we can't properly express, it's always a struggle just to survive. And it's this feeling of helplessness that sometimes drives us half crazy, and brings on a panic attack or a meltdown.
>
> (Higashida, 2007, p. 109)

The primary focus, then, of an intervention must be to instill a sense of safety in the child with autism, without which any kind of relational development or communication, whether verbal or nonverbal, would be extremely difficult to facilitate. A child with a high level of anxiety, who does not feel safe in the environment, is likely to shut down or close up in order to protect himself from perceived threat and pain inducing experiences.

Consider, for example, the first time Teo came for art therapy and his reluctance to enter the therapy room. Since Teo was unable to verbalise his apprehension, he communicated it physically through resistant body language and by staggering his entry. I reacted by letting Teo's mother into the therapy room with him for reassurance. Teo's reaction was reasonable considering he was in an unfamiliar environment and, faced with a stranger in my person, the unpredictability of the situation would have been a scary prospect for him. I allowed Teo's mother to sit through the therapy sessions until she could leave the room without any apparent distress to him. Teo was free to keep the door ajar if he so wished and could go in and out of the room at will to see his mother. Keeping in mind that "[i]n a safe environment, all children can move towards building a trusting relationship with a therapist" (Emery, 2002, p. 145), my foremost goal was to establish a sense of safety for Teo.

The therapist can get cues into the level of the child's anxiety by careful observation of his or her body language that may indicate a state of discomfort or relaxation, increase or decrease in self-stimulatory and rigid repetitive behaviors (RRBs), changes in vocalisations and resistance to entering the room among others. Below are some of the techniques I used to instill a sense of safety in my subjects.

Holding Back

In the first few sessions, Teo seemed uninterested in interacting with me or even in acknowledging my presence. I felt invisible in the room with him, especially when I actively tried to draw his attention by calling out his name, but there was no response. In the hope that perhaps art materials would evoke some curiosity in Teo, I laid them on the floor for easy access as opposed to a chair and table that could be more restrictive; however, Teo was not drawn to them. As mentioned earlier, Teo probably did not feel secure in a new environment and felt safer within himself instead of opening up to unfamiliar and unpredictable input. Considering Teo's mother had warned me of his lack of reciprocity, I should have been prepared for his aloof behavior, but I began to panic, possibly because I, too, did not feel safe with him, not knowing how he would respond to me, if at all. While Teo walked back and forth along one wall of the room, grazing it with his shoulder and singing nursery rhymes, not paying any attention to the art materials that I hoped would catch his attention, I moved on to playing drums and mimicking his songs. Teo remained oblivious to my overtures. Eventually, I began engaging with the art materials myself, learning to *hold back* or not engage actively with Teo until he was ready to interact with me on his own terms. The vignette below is from one of the earlier sessions that I had with Teo, in which I illustrate the practice of holding back.

Vignette 1

Teo followed me indifferently into the room. I walked to the center of the studio where I had laid out some art material on the floor. Teo stayed close to the wall nearest to the door and began to interweave vocalisations with lyrics from nursery rhymes. He walked along the side of the wall as he sang, touching it with his shoulders, then halting briefly to make small jerky movements with his hands. I called out to Teo, instinctively coaxing him to take note of the art material but he did not respond. I moved away from the art material and started to play the drum to draw his attention, banking on his affinity to music. The beat of the drum caught Teo's interest, and he ran toward me, or most likely the drum, not making any eye contact. He stayed in close proximity to me for a few seconds without attempting to touch the drum before running back to the wall. Perhaps he felt safer next to the wall and needed to touch base with it frequently. I continued beating the drum and added a nursery rhyme to it but Teo had lost interest. It was enough that Teo had noticed the drums and they had brought him closer to me even if for a short while. I abandoned the drum and let some time pass, *holding back* before approaching Teo, making sure I was at least an arm's length away from him. After I drew closer to him I began to mimic his songs and to mirror his body movements, especially the way he moved his hands. I was positioning myself as an attachment figure by attempting to share in his experience of sounds and movements. My actions elicited a glance from Teo and the fact that he had acknowledged my presence was a victory for me considering that he tended to show almost no interest in my existence. Upon receiving no further attention, I went back to the art materials that lay on the floor (holding back again) and began to dig out play dough from the different colored pots. My engagement with the play dough piqued Teo's attention, and he came towards me and sat down next to me. To my delight, Teo picked up one of the pots and began to take out the play dough from it before rolling it between his fingers.

The above vignette provides some insight into how the therapist can create a sense of safety for a child who might be closed up from the environment due to feelings of danger and high levels of anxiety stemming from sensory issues, unfamiliarity and unpredictability among others. The concept of holding back, or shifting between active engagement and reserve, may not be easy for a therapist who is eager for a response. It can also mean that a large part of the session may go without much activity or engagement between therapist and child in which the former may feel pressured to have something happen. However, the therapist must learn to be comfortable with periods of relative inactivity as that is what the child may need at that point in time in order to feel familiar and safe in the environment with them.

Making Art Yourself

During periods of holding back active engagement from Teo and Raj, I opted for what Martin (2009) called "acting as a live model" (p. 41), meaning I made art within sight of the boys but not in close proximity to them. Making art myself was not only an attempt to capture the boys' interest and motivate them to join me, it also helped me regulate my anxiety during the sessions

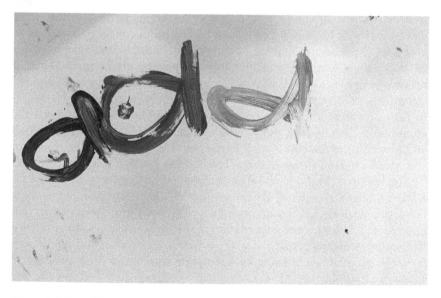

Figure 5.2 Raj: fish, paint on paper

when I felt uneasy with their lack of engagement. Thus, while Teo chose to keep to himself and Raj ran around the room stimming, seeking tactile input from paintbrushes that he held close to his chin, I made art with crayons drawing bright images of objects like cars, animals or plants likely to be familiar to the boys. At times I layered paper with paint spreading it with rollers to create striking patterns and images or used shaving foam to draw large circles on the mirror lined walls of the room using exaggerated movements with both arms. I found that some activities drew more interest from the boys than others. For instance, shaving foam almost always worked as a motivator to get the boys to approach me and engage with the foam, followed closely by pouring paint from a height to create patterns. More often than not, I complemented my actions with exaggerated vocalisations such as "oh, look at what I am making" or "this is so much fun" in order to create affect. Below I describe how I was able to motivate Raj for joint artmaking by first modeling for him and then using it as a platform for interaction.

Vignette 2

We were almost halfway through the 12 sessions. Raj entered the room and proceeded to grab the paintbrushes that he used as a stim object. Holding the brushes between both hands, their bristles touching his chin, Raj ran back and forth across the room as was his routine. I sat on the floor with bottles of paint and sheets of paper and began to draw shapes, observing Raj for any cues of his desire to connect. Raj remained aloof. After some time, I called out his name, hopeful he would look my way. To my delight, upon hearing his name, Raj ran up to me, picked up a brush, dipped it in paint and made a brisk mark across the paper. Before I could express my amazement at his overture or do anything to prolong his engagement, Raj threw the brush on the sheet and ran back to the other end of the room before resorting to his stimming. Optimistic that what had worked once may work yet again, I called Raj a second time. He responded, and this time when he held the brush, I guided his stroke to make a shape. The shape that was created resembled a fish and I immediately pointed to the image and named it "fish" hoping to sustain Raj's interest (see Figure 5.2). Unexpectedly Raj repeated the word "fish" after me and sat long enough for me to quickly draw three stick figures. I named them "boy," "Huma" and "mummy," pointing to each respectively. Raj repeated the words "boy" and "Huma" and I praised him effusively before he moved away. This was the first time Raj, who had very limited expressive language, had repeated words after me and associated them with marks on paper. Our interaction, though brief, had been meaningful. The session gave me some insight into Raj's developmental level and his ability to engage when suitably motivated. It helped to reaffirm my faith in taking things slowly and not to get impatient for results.

Approach, Engage and Retreat

The concepts of *holding back* and *making art oneself* tie in in with the *approach engage and retreat* technique that Evans and Dubowski (2001) proposed to build up tolerance to eventually move closer to the child. I found that with Alex, an approach, engage and retreat technique at certain times in the sessions worked especially well, as illustrated through the vignette.

Vignette 3

When Alex said he did not want to come into the art therapy room, I left him in the waiting area with his mother and went back into the room. Alex followed soon after. This sequence of events had become a pattern. I had learnt that if I insisted Alex come into the room he would likely resist. Hence, an approach, engage and retreat technique worked best with him. Alex had already had a few sessions of art therapy with me, and according to his mother liked coming for them. I had a similar impression of Alex since he seemed to enjoy artmaking, especially engaging with his favorite materials: paints and kinetic sand. Hence, it could be assumed that his resistance to enter the room was reflective of difficulty with transition or/and was his way of exerting control rather than a dislike of the intervention itself. My nonchalant attitude toward Alex's refusal to join me in the room diminished the chance of a confrontation with him, additionally allowing him the space to bring about a shift in his oppositional behavior and enter the room on his own terms.

Subsequently, Alex came into the room and picked up a rubber caterpillar. He began pulling and tugging at it and I joined him (approach) in playing with the caterpillar, before showing him the face paints that I had bought for him. In earlier sessions, Alex had rubbed paint-laden hands on his face and I thought he would enjoy using face paints; however, his response to this new material was lukewarm. Consequently, I directed him to sand play, one of his favorite activities, where Alex and I filled moulds with kinetic sand to construct buildings (engage). Though Alex enjoyed sand play, his attention span was short, and I usually had a line-up of activities that I could direct him to in quick succession to prolong his cycle of engagement with me. Hence, after the sand play, I guided him to a table where he could paint. From past experience, I was conscious that paint was likely to induce hyperarousal in Alex, especially as his engagement with it increased in length. I expected Alex's capacity to self-regulate would be tested, and I had guessed correctly. Alex poured paint onto the paper from the squeeze bottles and began to layer it with the rollers. For him the ritual of mixing the colors and the process of applying them seemed to be more meaningful than the marks that he was making. Alex seemed engrossed in the act when suddenly, he dipped his fingers in the paint and proceeded to rub them all over his face as if it was a most gratifying experience. I am not sure whether it was the sensation of the paint on his face that he liked or a release that the act provided him, but I was reluctant to let him use the paints on his face lest they enter his eyes (hence I had procured the face paints). Therefore, I feigned an alarmed expression and showed concern about the paint going into Alex's eyes before accompanying him to the toilet to wash the paint off. After returning to the room, I decided not to engage Alex directly since our prior interaction had been intense and full of action (retreat). Thus, I pretended to explore the basket of toys that lay on a table across the room some distance away from Alex who wandered around the room. I moved on from the toy basket to scribbling with crayons on paper. This drew Alex's attention and he joined me in playing scribble tag (engage). The session was coming to a close, and I indicated it was time for Alex to go home. Suddenly, Alex grabbed the caterpillar he had been playing with earlier and ran to the table at the far end of the room and sat under it refusing to come out. My coaxing and cajoling fell on deaf ears and I once again I decided to retreat from interaction. I moved on to the mirrored wall and began to draw on it with glass markers. As I had anticipated, my lack of reaction and Alex's motivation to use the markers drew him out from under the table. After drawing with the markers, Alex was able to let go of the caterpillar and head home.

Body Positioning

Evans and Dubowski (2001) have identified other aspects of therapy that contribute toward the sense of safety in the child. Apart from the gauging the *approach retreat sensitivity* of the child, they advise careful attention to the body positioning of the therapist in relation to the child. They recommend an *invitation position*, where the level of the therapist is at or below the child's level with the head tilted to one side and limited eye contact and language. With Teo and Raj, I conducted most of the sessions on the floor where I was at level with them. I felt this made me less threatening and also allowed them to move freely around me and the art materials. With Alex I used both the floor and the small table and chair, which kept me at level with him. Evans and Dubowski (2001) mentioned that moving too quickly or too closely with one of their clients evoked a violent response. Cognizant of the importance of body space, throughout their sessions I was conscious of the distance be-tween myself and the boys, not wanting to invade their body space in order to maintain their sense of safety.

Indicators That the Child May Be Feeling Safe

a) The child enters the room willingly and does not object to the door being closed.
b) The child does not attempt to leave the room frequently.
c) There is no undue increase in stimming or RRBs.

d) The child is comfortable with the therapist approaching him or her and with close proximity to the latter.
e) The child initiates proximity to or contact with the therapist.
f) Other indicators may be increase in eye contact and reciprocal behaviors such as listening to directives, turn taking, sharing art materials and so on.

Tips

a) Pre-empt the child's level of anxiety by observing increase in overt behaviors.
b) Do not force the child to enter the room. Allow the caregiver to sit in or keep the door ajar during the sessions.
c) Do not seek to actively engage the child. Give the child time and space to become familiar.
d) Make art yourself using attractive materials to motivate the child to initiate contact.
e) Be comfortable with breaks and pauses in the session.
f) Gauge when to approach, engage and retreat from the child. Learn to sit with inactivity if that is what it takes to make the child feel safe.
g) Pay attention to your own body language and positioning in relation to the child.

Conclusion

Creating a sense of safety is one of the foremost and perhaps the most critical elements of the therapy sessions for a child with ASD who may be predisposed to high anxiety caused by the challenges inherent in the spectrum. Maintaining the sense of safety requires a switched on, sensitive and attuned therapist who is able to pre-empt anxiety provoking situations and assess fluctuations in anxiety levels throughout the session. A child who feels safe with the therapist will be more open and receptive to engagement than one who is fearful and apprehensive and shuts down to defend against feelings of danger.

References

Durrani, H. (2019). Art therapy's scope to address attachment in children with ASD and comorbid SID. *Journal of Art Therapy*. 10.1080/07421656.2019.1677063.
Emery, M. J. (2002). Art therapy as an intervention for autism. *Art Therapy: Journal of the American Art Therapy Association*, 2(3), 143–147. https://doi.org/10.1080/07421656.2004.10129500.
Evans, K., & Dubowski, J. (2001). *Art therapy with children on the autistic spectrum*. London, England: Jessica Kingsley.
Higashida, N. (2007). *The reason I jump*. New York: NY: Random House.
Martin, N. (2009). *Art as an early intervention tool for children with autism*. London, England: Jessica Kingsley.

6   Sensory Regulation

In the chapter that covers sensory integration dysfunction (SID), I detailed the different kinds of sensory regulation issues that children on the spectrum may face and how each child has a unique sensory profile. Whatever the child's sensory profile, the art therapist must thoroughly familiarise him- or herself with it before commencing therapy in order to avoid unintentional discomfort to the child. Details of a child's sensory hypo- and hypersensitivities may be accessible through occupational therapy reports or a discussion with the child's caregiver. Where possible, ongoing consultation with the child's occupational therapist is a good idea to keep abreast of any developments or changes in the child's sensory profile. A quote taken from Greenspan and Wieder's book, = *Engaging Autism*, relates directly to the theme of sensory regulation in the S-BRATA, "To help children be comfortable in the world, clinicians and caregivers must first learn by careful observation which sensations help children become calm and regulated, which ones overwhelm them, and which don't pull them in enough. Whatever the infant or child's age, you the caregiver need to observe how she responds to different types of touch on different parts of her body. Experiment with different sounds—high- and low-pitched noises, the normal human voice—and different degrees of volume to see which ones draw the child's attention more. Do this with each of the senses. This helps you determine which senses to emphasise as you draw the child into your world" (Greenspan & Wieder, 2006, p. 73).

Teo, Raj and Alex had a varied sensory profile with hypo- and hypersensitivities across multiple domains. For instance, they were all tactile seeking, but the intensity of their needs differed from each other. Alex required much heavier tactile input compared to Teo and Raj, indicating greater tactile and proprioceptive needs, whereas the latter sought significantly more movement than the other two boys, pointing to an under-responsive vestibular system. Fortunately, for me, having lived with Moeez, I had exposure to a spectrum of sensory impairments and although each child has a unique sensory profile, the anxiety stemming from a discordant sensory system may manifest in similar behaviors. For example, Teo was not responsive to his name when I first saw him and I had experienced the same situation with Moeez as a child.

Although it is very possible that the causality of the behavior in both children emanated from disparate sensory issues, the symptom was similar. Stated another way, my experience with Moeez alerted me to Teo's probable underlying sensory needs, and I was careful not to attribute his lack of response to absence of interest to engage with me.

Before I began sessions with Teo, Raj and Alex, I interviewed their caregivers in a preliminary meeting where I gathered anecdotal evidence of their sensory needs as no occupational therapy reports were available. Hence, I did not have access to professional insight into their sensory profile, which would have helped further my understanding of their needs. However, I keenly observed the boys for overt behaviors that confirmed their caregivers' account of their sensory profile. The following sub-themes lie under the umbrella of the overarching theme of *sensory regulation* and are illustrated through vignettes.

Observation and Anticipation

As mentioned before, the themes of the S-BRATA are not sequential in nature and run concurrent to each other. Therefore, it is not possible to work with any one theme in isolation as they are closely linked to each other. Hence, both the themes of *safety* and *sensory regulation* must run hand in hand as the absence of one may become the source of the other. The therapist can achieve this concurrent process through prior knowledge of the child's sensory profile followed by a keen sense of observation in the session. The cognizant therapist must look out for signs of anxiety in the child that may be indicated by increase in restricted repetitive behaviors (RRBs), stimming, the child's body posture (whether relaxed or tense) and loud vocalisations, among others. The following vignette will illustrate how observation and anticipation can guide the therapist's sense of direction in regulating the child.

Vignette 1

Alex had a propensity to grind his teeth in order to compensate for the lack of proprioceptive input he sought. During one particular session, he entered the therapy room grinding his teeth excessively. The teeth grinding, coupled with a tense posture and restless body language, indicated that Alex was highly anxious. I was alerted to the possibility that Alex may dysregulate easily and prepared myself mentally to handle the outcome. Typically, Alex asked to use paints, his favorite medium, and I would allow him, but that day observing his uneasy state, I directed him toward sand play. Alex was familiar with the sand and mold activity and had enjoyed it in previous sessions. Handling the sand and packing the molds tightly with it provided him with heavy tactile input that grounded him. I hoped it would have the same calming effect in this session. To enhance the impact of Alex's engagement with the sand, I devised a game where I asked Alex to first make the molds and then break them by pounding his fists. Alex was delighted to undertake this kung-fu act and proceeded to flatten the sculptures with both fists exuberantly. He asked to repeat this sequence of making and breaking the molds many times. Alex's teeth grinding lessened and eventually stopped during the sand play. His body posture relaxed and I sensed his anxiety levels come down. I could then direct him to using his favorite medium, paint.

Practicing Self-Regulation

We live in a world bombarded with sensory input from the environment. Whether they are sounds, sights, smells or textures, our sensory system is constantly processing information through our sensory organs. For those of us with a relatively healthy sensory system, we do this relatively effortlessly. However, for children with SID, the same system that neurotypicals take for granted can be a source of great anxiety. Although the environment can sometimes be modified to facilitate the child with SID, it is not always possible to do so. For instance, schools can allocate a quiet corner in the classroom for overwhelmed children or caregivers can provide sound-canceling headphones to their young ones in loud places such as supermarkets; however, sometimes unwelcome sensory input from the environment may be unavoidable. Ideally, if the child is taught to self-regulate, he or she would be better equipped to deal with anxiety-provoking stimuli. In my work with Alex and Teo, I found that cycles of inducing and reducing arousal levels were a good way of practising self-regulation, reminiscent of the co-regulatory activity between mother and child. One way of achieving this is by moving between art materials with contrasting affect while managing highs and lows as explicated in the following vignette.

Vignette 2

In the same session as the preceding vignette, once Alex was better regulated after the sand play and his teeth grinding had stopped, I directed him to use paint in order to alternate a modulating activity with a stimulating one that was likely to cause a rise in his arousal levels. I chose a palette with small but deep indents to provide Alex with a visual cue to control the amount of paint he poured out, pairing it with an auditory prompt to "stop" when the paint reached the rim of the indent. In previous sessions where I had given Alex a flat palette or when he poured paint directly on to the paper, he would quickly squeeze out large amounts of the material, triggering a sudden escalation in excitement. Cognizant of the rousing effect of paint on Alex, I attempted to slow down the process of arousal by encouraging him to use sponge cut-outs for stamping rather than using a paintbrush or rollers (see Figure 6.1). Stamping and dabbing paint with sponges is a relatively contained activity since sponge absorbs a fair amount of the paint before it can be applied onto the paper, as opposed to a

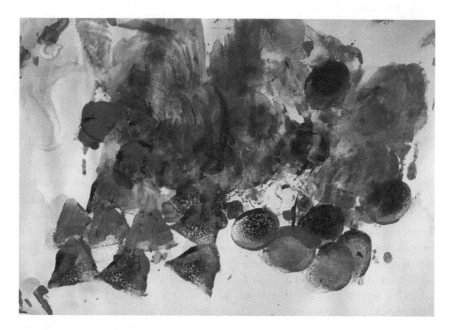

Figure 6.1   Alex: stamping with sponges

brush or roller, which are more freeing. Also, the motion of dabbing and pressing the sponge onto a hard surface requires heavier proprioception compared to the more fluid movements of brushwork. Alex began to stamp the paper with the sponges but gradually the excitement of using paint gained momentum and he moved on to stamping his arms and then his face. Next, he rose and began to stamp the mirrored wall alternating between his face and the mirror. Alex had reached a state of higher arousal compared to the sand play, and before he could dysregulate further, I directed him away from the paint to punching stamps that had to be pressed really hard to generate paper cut-outs. I anticipated that the effort that Alex would have to put into the motion of pressing the stamps would provide him sufficient proprioceptive input to induce calm and lower his excitement level. The punching activity helped Alex settle down and he spent a considerable amount of time doing it. The switch from sand to paint to stamping was done intentionally to induce low and high arousal in Alex. The idea was to aid the internalisation of self-regulation through repeated cycles of alternating affect.

Being Comfortable with Unpredictability

Greenspan & Wieder (2006) stated, "[C]hildren show us their own solutions to their sensory processing system challenges. It's up to us to recognize the solution and figure out a way to expand on it by making it interactive. For example, an under reactive child who is lying on her tummy and pushing a car back and forth is seeking support from the floor. To engage her, lie down on the floor in front of her, and, as she pushes the car around aimlessly, you can either meet her with another car, crash your car into hers, or push it further away. Once she's engaged and begins to get more mobilized, you can start moving her up the ladder, using her sensory needs to guide the interactions" (p. 144). I agree with Greenspan that the children themselves give cues to what they need from the intervention, whether it is communicated verbally or through explicit behaviors. However, there are times that the therapist may get thrown by unforeseen reactions and unpredictable outcomes. It can be that a particular art material has a certain effect one day and the next time it is used it evokes a contradictory response. Hence, the therapist who is expecting to ground a child through play dough may end up with the same child eating the material and dysregulating instead. I have been in a such a situation with a 7-year-old where I ended up battling the child to prevent them from choking on the clay they had mouthed. Similarly with Raj, I struggled to regulate him at times, as he had a tendency to escalate into high arousal faster than I could anticipate. Below is brief illustration of an unforeseen interaction with Raj.

Vignette 3

Since Raj had shown little interest in paint and crayons, I had prepared a large ball of bright blue goop for him to motivate him with something more novel than traditional art materials. Instead of approaching Raj directly, I began to play with the goop while he wandered around the room. I stretched and pulled the goop voicing my enjoyment as I played with it. I was delighted when my engagement with the material immediately drew his attention and he came toward me and took some of the goop from my hands and began to pull at it, vocalizing as he did so. I mirrored Raj's actions and mimicked his expression in an attempt to draw him into joint play. For a few seconds it seemed my plan had worked when Raj and I connected through mutual tugging and pulling of the goop, when suddenly Raj became very animated and started running around the room with the material, laughing and vocalizing loudly. He began to break off pieces of the goop and throw them on the floor jumping excitably and vocalizing even louder. I was thrown off by Raj's behavior and had to take the goop away from him before he ended up walking all over it and pasting it on to the floor. Although I had managed to catch Raj's attention with a different art material, I did not anticipate the resulting high arousal. I was uncertain whether it was the texture of the goop or something else that had triggered Raj's arousal, and I had to sit with the discomfort of not knowing. I was disappointed by the result of my attempt since it had been very difficult to motivate Raj with traditional art materials and his attention to the goop had given me hope. I felt both physically and mentally challenged with the unpredictability of

Raj's response and had to learn to manage my expectations from him as well as myself.

Conclusion

A dysregulated child is an anxious child who is having a hard time dealing with the outside world. Facilitating regulation in the child is analogous to making him or her feel safe and less anxious. The therapist must have as much detail as possible of the sensory profile of the child before starting therapy and through its duration, develop a deeper understanding of the child's behaviors and responses through constant observation and anticipation. Self-regulation can be practiced and instilled in the child through interchanging art materials that evoke complementary responses. Even so, things may not go according to plan in some sessions, and that is not unusual nor should it be a reason for beating yourself up. Unpredictability is part of the process of working with children with autism, and it is important to give yourself time to work through ups and downs and adapt to changing probabilities.

Tips

a) Familiarise yourself with the child's sensory profile before starting therapy.
b) Observe the child for increase in RRBs, self-stimulatory behaviors and variations in that may indicate an escalation of anxiety.
c) Don't be afraid to experiment with different materials to gauge their effect on the child.
d) Alternate between high and low arousal to practice self-regulation.
e) Anticipate unpredictable outcomes and learn to be comfortable with them.
f) Manage your expectations.

Reference

Greenspan, S. I. & Wieder, S. (2006). *Engaging autism (a Merloyd Lawrence book)* (Kindle Edition). Philadelphia, PA: Da Capo Press.

7 Mirroring and Attunement

The layered communication between mother and child is in part instinctual and part intentional, where through the choreography of the social exchange, the child learns about himself and the outside world (Stern, 1977). "Recognition is that response from the other which makes meaningful the feelings, intentions, and actions of the self" (Benjamin, 1988 p. 12). The idea or concept of recognition by *another*, also referred to as a *subject* by the intersubjective theorists, is personified through the attachment relationship, epitomised through the mutually instinctive identification and response between caregiver and child that is mediated through reciprocal attachment behaviors.

Stern (1977) detailed his observation of the mother-infant early social interaction in the following passage where he described the intricate exchange between the dyad during the process of breast feeding:

> The mother turned her head and gazed at the infant's face. He was gazing at the ceiling, but out of the corner of his eye he saw her head turn toward him and turned to gaze back at her. This had happened before but now he broke rhythm and stopped sucking. He let go of the nipple and the suction around it broke as he eased into the faintest suggestion of a smile. The mother abruptly stopped talking and, as she watched his face begin to transform, her eyes opened a little wider and her eyebrows raised a bit. His eyes locked on to hers, and together they held motionless for an instant. The infant did not turn to sucking and his mother held frozen her slight expression of anticipation. The silent and almost motionless instant continued to hang until the mother suddenly shattered it by saying "Hey!" and simultaneously opening her eyes wider, raising her eyebrows further and throwing her head up and toward the infant. (p. 18)

Mirroring or reflecting back and *attunement* or being in synch with another are the fundamental attachment behaviors that underpin the caregiver-child interactions and have been beautifully illustrated in the above example through the harmonious reciprocity between the mother and child. Wright (2009), too, explained it within the context of the mother-child relationship in which the former responds "in a moment by moment way, to the smaller changes of excitement and arousal that accompany everything the baby does" (called by Stern the *vitality affects*). The mother tracks these smaller changes as we track a tennis player during an exciting game – she reads her baby by every possible nonverbal means and intuitively senses the changing pattern of his feeling state: the contours of arousal, the rhythms of excitement, the urgent strivings and triumphant satisfactions (p. 67). This kind of tuning in or mutual resonance between two individuals is consonant with feeling of *einfuhlung* or flow (Csikszentmihalyi, 1990) that emanate from embodied experiences or "body-centered intelligence" (Kossak, 2009, p. 14). Essentially, this intersubjective experience mediated through sensory and perceptual experiences, which results in a "deep shared connectivity" (Kossak, 2009, P. 16), is also referred to as *entrainment* (Thaut, Kenyon, Schauer, & McIntosh, 1999) and *vicarious introspection*.

I have iterated before that concurrent to addressing sensory integration dysfunction (SID) in children with autism, the S-BRATA aims to foster an attachment relationship between therapist and child. Due to the high frequency of qualitative differences in attachment patterns of children with ASD that point to possible impairments, an attachment relationship with the therapist has positive implications for the psycho-emotional development of the child, especially since an old, unhealthy pattern of attachment can be replaced by a new, healthier one.

Arts-based interventions that take a mind-body approach entail "the kind of mutual resonance experienced as connectivity, unity, understanding, support, empathy and acceptance, that can contribute greatly to creating a sense of psychological healing" (Kossak, 2009). Due to the multimodal and visceral nature of such interventions, they are ideally suited for attachment work that emanates from *embodied intelligence* (Kossak, 2009) or the ability of the body and mind to experience the world in a meaningful way, asserting the intercorporeal nature of existing in the world (Merleau-Ponty, 1962). Referring to attunement within the expressive arts, Kossak (2015) stated that it "includes awareness of breath, movement, impulses, sensation, and associative emotions, and can be linked directly to psychological states of being" (p. 37). He seems to be referring to a state of attuned consciousness and subconsciousness that is both physiological and emotional; a subliminal intelligence that underpins the in-synch relationship.

Mirror Neuron System (MNS)

In the past couple of decades, there has been considerable interest in the relationship between the arts and science. The upsurge in neuroscientific research has yielded fascinating evidence of a neurobiological basis for mirroring through the discovery of the mirror neuron system (MNS) that I have briefly discussed in chapter 3. The MNS has important implications for mind-body based interventions as it suggests that an individual's actions, intentions and feelings are literally reflected in the brain of the person looking at them. Thus, for the therapist-child dyad, where the end goal is the formation of an attachment, the act of mirroring may contribute significantly toward the phenomena of therapeutic attunement and embodied intelligence. Moreover, studies have shown an impairment in the MNS of individuals with autism (Gallese, 2005; Oberman, Pineda, & Ramachandaran, 2007), and coupled with the lack of theory of mind (TOM) or the ability to relate to another person's psychoemotional state, the impairment in the MNS may exacerbate the relational challenges inherent in the spectrum. Importantly, however, research points to the possibility of the enhancement of the MNS in children with autism through positive relational experiences (Warren et al., 2006). This has positive implications for the development of the MNS of children with ASD. Hence, it may be argued that mirroring or reflecting back to the child with ASD not only promotes attachment, it may also have a positive impact on the development of the MNS.

The following vignettes illustrate the phenomena of mirroring and attunement through three successive sessions with Teo. I have attempted to describe the explicit and implicit processes that underpinned my interaction with Teo with the goal of forming an attachment with him; however, it was simply impossible to capture in words the minute-to-minute movements, sensations, impulses and emotions that facilitated a kind of deep connectivity and attuned consciousness.

It is important to remember that the themes of the S-BRATA run parallel to each other and are not meant to be implemented in stages. Therefore, at the same time as I focused on attuning to Teo, I was equally conscious of maintaining a sense of safety and addressing his sensory needs.

Vignette 1

Teo routinely perseverated on nursery rhymes that he sang as he walked and sometimes ran around the room. His mother shared that he had probably learnt the rhymes from watching videos at home. Teo's continuous singing seemed to play the role of a regulatory mechanism that kept Teo safe inside his world and his constant movement in the room pointed to sensory seeking behavior, possibly arising from an impairment in the vestibular domain. Not wanting to disrupt Teo's routine behaviors that were obviously serving some purpose, I decided to join him by mimicking those behaviors with the purpose of maintaining a sense of safety by not forcing him to stop and pay attention to me. Also, I felt I did not know Teo enough to push his boundaries and did not feel safe enough with him in the first few sessions as I had not developed the kind of connectivity that enables the embodied work that leads to an attuned reciprocity. Hence, I ran around the room with Teo pretending to play tag, validating his actions even when he did not seem to be paying attention to me. I mimicked his vocalisations hoping he might respond if I could give meaning to his utterances through "protoconversations ('motherese')," as described by Evans and Dubowski (2001, p. 50). Therefore, when Teo sang, I sang along with him and followed his movements, keeping a safe distance. In the first few sessions, my attempts were met with sidelong glances from Teo interspersed with brief pauses in his singing. Unsure of what these intermissions meant, I was happy to see that he was beginning to notice me through fleeting glances in my direction. Even the smallest reaction from Teo was an endorsement to persevere and be patient with the pace of progress. As the sessions went on, I became increasingly comfortable just being around Teo. Whereas in the beginning sessions, there were frequent instances of frustration and a sense of urgency for something to happen, I gradually settled into a more acquiescent frame of mind. Finally, in session nine, there was a sudden shift In Teo's behavior and to my amazement he responded for the first time to his name. I had been playing with shaving foam some distance away from him following the approach and retreat technique that I have described in chapter 5 under the theme of sense of safety, when Teo walked up to me. Although his interaction was fleeting, in that he did not engage with me beyond moving in my direction, he had approached me instead of the other way around. This was after eight sessions where I had initiated most of the interactions and Teo had only acknowledged my existence through glances. Teo's reaction to his name was even more remarkable because, according to his mother, he would not even respond to her when called. It seemed that something had happened through the last eight sessions that had allowed Teo to venture out of his inner world and communicate with the outside. There could be multiple reasons why Teo made the jump from his inner world to the environment: possibly he felt safe within a space where he could set the pace and there was no expectation to perform, maybe he felt validated by my consistent mirroring and was motivated to respond or my increased sense of ease with Teo was indicative of a mutual understanding and acceptance.

This small victory with Teo was just one of the highlights of the session because later on, Teo made another huge leap in communication when he filled in the gaps of the alphabet that I was singing. This happened a few times and I noticed during this cycle of engagement Teo's eye contact with me increased as well. Rather than the cursory glances I had received earlier, Teo seemed to be *seeing* me. It reminded me of the *recognition* that Benjamin (1988) talked about that gives meaning to the existence of the other person or the mutually instinctive identification that underpins the attachment relationship. Our unconventional conversation was a turning point in Teo's therapy as henceforth Teo and my interactions gained further impetus.

Vignette 2

Teo looked at me from time to time as I sat on the floor painting. He walked around the room singing as was his routine. I joined him in his song and called out to him to come sit with me. Teo came over and sat right opposite me across the paper I was painting on. He did not attempt to touch the art material; instead, he turned to the mirror-lined wall and made a face. I caught his eyes in the mirror and copied him in a playful manner. I hoped that our mirror neurons were firing away. Next, Teo stood up and walked to a corner of the room and I followed him mimicking his vocalisations. I grabbed a marker from a nearby table and made a mark on Teo's hand. I was now comfortable in close proximity to him and felt I could take the liberty to establish physical contact. Teo did not seem to mind my overture. I returned to the art material on the floor since I did not want to overwhelm Teo with too much close interaction and added shaving foam to the paint, estimating it would attract him. I was looking for Teo to initiate contact on his own terms. The shaving foam caught Teo's attention, and he joined me on the floor and began to touch the foam. Teo mumbled something that sounded like the color *green*, and I immediately repeated the word after him to give meaning to his vocalisation. Teo's ensuing action confirmed the accuracy of my estimation when Teo put some blue paint on his hand saying the word *blue* followed by *pink*. I pointed to pink paint bottle repeating the word *pink*. The length that Teo's functional communication had come in such a short span of time was incredible. It was almost as if a portal had opened to another universe and Teo was taking the first steps into it. After that, Teo got up to wander around the room, and I did not follow him, allowing him space to be by himself. It was sufficient that a palpable connection had been made between us: now it was my turn to step back and let Teo set the pace of engagement between us. I squeezed some more shaving foam onto the paper, suspecting that Teo would be drawn to it again, and I was rewarded when Teo joined me again and this time around spread the shaving foam onto the paper. I praised him enthusiastically and continued to mirror his vocalisations as if it were a conversation that we were having. Sensing Teo's level of comfort in this session I dabbed my finger in some paint and asked for Teo's hand. When he directed his hand towards me, I marked it with paint. Since Teo did not object, I kept on adding different colours to his hand and transitioned from painting on the back of the hand to turning it over and circling his palm with my finger. As I circled his palm, I began to sing, "Round and round the garden Like a Teddy Bear; one step, two step tickle under there" (a rhyme that accompanies fingerplay in which the adult draws light circles on the child's palm before walking their index and middle figure up the elbow and toward the shoulder to tickle under the arm). Teo stopped his own singing to listen to me and appeared to enjoy the play. The entire exchange left me feeling overwhelmingly like a mother who had bonded with her child through touch, gesture and harmonious interaction in a *moment by moment way* described by Wright (2009). Something special had passed between Teo and me in that session.

Vignette 3

Between this session and the last, Teo was away for one week. When I met Teo's mother before the session, she was very excited to share that Teo had been trying to approach and imitate other children in the park. He had never done this before, and she felt he was opening up and noticing his environment. I was equally excited to learn of Teo's progress, and recalling the previous session, I hoped this session would bring up even more opportunities to extend my length of engagement with him. I began the session by making art myself and mirroring Teo's vocalisations as per usual. I drew the letter A saying it out loud to catch Teo's interest. Teo wandered around the room and did not pay attention. I then picked up a bottle of paint and from some height dripped some of it on the paper accompanying my action with exaggerated affect. Teo looked my way but still did not approach me. Finally, it was the shaving foam that did the trick again, and Teo came over and began to spread the foam on the paper. While Teo engaged with the foam, I dripped paint on it forming different patterns to keep Teo motivated to engage with the artmaking. During this interplay of foam and paint, Teo walked away a few times and returned to the art engaging briefly with the foam while I continued playing with the foam and paint mimicking his vocalisations on and off. A while later, when Teo lay on the floor, I joined him and he allowed me to draw circles on his hand with paint. Once again I sang "Round and Round the Garden" and traced circles on Teo's hands. Teo appeared to be enjoying the experience and the length of our engagement increased as I improvised the fingerplay by dipping my fingers in different colors of paint and drawing circles with them. Teo appeared to be very relaxed and I stopped the play wanting to see his reaction and that is when he put his hand forward indicating that he wanted me to continue.

The session above was Teo's second last. It was bittersweet for me because I felt he was opening up beautifully and responding with increased motivation. Unfortunately I had to stop as the 12 sessions allocated to the research were over. However, Teo's progress through the sessions and his mother's positive feedback were heartwarming. Before I said goodbye to Teo in the last session, I flung a soft ball at him and he threw it back at me, responding as any other child would in a game of catch. Teo couldn't have left me with a better farewell gift.

Rupture and Repair

Attunement and misattunement or rupture and repair are part of any attachment relationship. Many such instances occur during caregiver-child interactions in which each may feel out of synch with the other on occasion only to re-establish the bond by riding out the storm. Though the rupture may be upsetting, it is the repair that follows after that validates the strength of the relationship. Especially for the child, the pattern of rupture and repair repeated multiple times teaches fearlessness from disappointment and instills trust in relationships.

Therefore, the therapist who is also positioned as an attachment figure need not consider rupture in the therapy session a failure; rather, it is an opportunity to establish a stronger relationship, provided the misattunement is addressed. In session eight with Alex, I had the occasion to experience an instance of rupture where he indulged in disruptive behavior that resulted in me having to cut short the session. The intensity of his tantrum and refusal to calm down left me with no other option but to manage his outburst by putting firm boundaries around him (I have narrated this incident in more detail under the theme of structure and boundaries in chapter 9). Although the following session was less chaotic, it continued to feel dissonant and ended up in another tantrum toward the end. I addressed Alex's behavior with consistent boundary setting, and eventually he responded by settling down. According to Kossak, "In expressive arts therapy this misattunement can lead a client to feel uncared for and unsupported, and can trigger deeper feelings of betrayal, or abuse. However, misattunement may be an important and necessary stage of psychological development, if a safe environment can be established where a re-experiencing of mistuned moments allows for new awareness, a shift in consciousness, and where new actions and reactions can be integrated" (p. 16). In Alex's case, it was not that he felt unsafe; however, it is possible that he was testing my boundaries to gauge my support for him. Hence, I had to carefully balance my response toward him by ensuring my empathy and acceptance but also by communicating my expectations of Alex's behavior.

Countertransference and Self-Awareness

The therapist's feelings of countertransference, or emotional reaction toward the child, are as much a window into themselves as they are into the child. In fact, self-awareness is an indispensable tool that the therapist can use to preempt, plan and adjust the intervention as and when required. For instance, I realised that I was susceptible to Alex's charm, especially when he praised me, "Huma you are wearing a nice shirt," beaming a big smile or resisted leaving the session because he liked it so much. I was tempted to believe that Alex's refusal to go home meant he would miss me, when in reality Alex had difficulty with transitioning from one place to another as well as a tendency to push boundaries. Had I not taken note of the feelings that I was projecting on Alex, I may have struggled with maintaining boundaries in the sessions that he certainly required. Similarly, with Raj, I struggled with feelings of frustration and at times annoyance when he showed a lack of motivation and resistance toward engaging with me. It took a lot of effort to overcome my countertransference with Raj, a sense of rejection that I felt from him, for me to remain invested in the sessions. Where Teo was concerned, my transference was overwhelmingly of a mother wanting to protect her child, and hence my interaction with him was imbued with a lot of patience and *motherese* (Evans & Dubowski, 2001).

Nevertheless, it can be difficult to constantly stay alert through the duration of the session, but the importance of self-awareness cannot be emphasised enough. I found that my bodily reactions and the ability to read subtle signals from them were a crucial source of information about the relational dynamics of the session. For example, I sensed that my level of anxiety would escalate when one of the boys was feeling anxious in the session. For instance, when Alex was grinding his teeth excessively in one session, I felt his tension in my chest and abdomen as I sat opposite him trying to engage him in sand play. As Alex calmed down and his teeth grinding reduced, I felt my body relax as well. Similarly, other somatic re-actions such as increase in heart rate, bodily tension or discomfort provide valuable insight into the direction the session may be going. I tried as much as I could to pay attention to my bodily responses and often caught myself clenching my jaw or talking excessively when things did not go as anticipated or I felt stuck. In the first few sessions with Teo, I felt I was vocalising nonstop to fill up the silence in the sessions. When I became aware of my tendency, I consciously reminded myself to hold back until I became com-fortable with the quiet periods in the sessions.

Body Language/Positioning

The body language, body positioning, facial expressions and tone of voice of the therapist have an impact on how they are perceived by the child. These attri-butes contribute to the feeling of safety and comfort that are prerequisite for any intervention. Thus, the therapist should embody a warm and welcoming attitude without being too effusive and try to be as consistent as possible since un-predictability can throw off the child with autism. Henley (2018) cited the case of Ebie who, despite immense neglect (Ebie was locked in a cellar during the day for five years, resulting in animalistic behaviors) and very limited interactions, began to warm up to the art therapy intern. He suggested that the intern's "smiling face, with a smooth, rounded female form, might have contributed to reopening a missed tactile and visual developmental window" (p. 117).

I usually like to meet children in the waiting room with a cheerful greeting before showing them the way to the room. Some children walk in immediately while others may require a bit more time and encouragement. Sometimes I bring out toys or art materials to motivate children to come into the room, as I did for Alex. I mentioned earlier that the caregiver is welcome to enter with the child and sit in the session until the child is at ease being alone in the room with me, as in Teo's case.

In the beginning sessions, I consciously maintain some distance from the children unless they initiate proximity or I sense they are comfortable with me coming closer to them. During my sessions with Teo and Raj, I mostly sat with the art materials on a plastic sheet laid on the floor. Fortunately, my studio has rubber flooring, which makes for comfortable sitting. I felt that with me on the floor, I would appear less threatening to the children, and it allowed them more postural flexibility where they could choose to sit or lie down beside me or opposite me. For Alex, I used both the floor and a children's table and chairs as he required less movement than the other two boys.

Tone of Voice

I tend to use a slightly high-pitched tone of voice with children who are resistant to engage, require motivation or encouragement. With children who are hyper-aroused, I am inclined to make use of a deeper, softer but firm tone. Hence with Teo and Raj, I employed exaggerated affect to direct their attention to me, whereas with Alex, I mostly used a lower tone of voice to keep him grounded and establish a sense of control when I felt that he may dysregulate. I can safely attribute my training in using a specific tone of voice to my having spent the past two decades raising a child with autism who had severe communication challenges and his share of tantrums and challenging behaviors.

Conclusion

The phenomena of mirroring and attunement underpin implicit and explicit attachment behaviors between therapist and child in which the former is positioned as the attachment figure. Central to these behaviors is the therapist's sensitivity to the affective state of the child, and that may be reflected in the somatic experience of the therapist. The therapist's ability to connect with the child at their level, on their terms, whether it is through play, music or protoconversations, is critical to opening up the child for communication and motivating him or her to initiate engagement. Instances of countertransference are opportunities for learning and insight into the relationship that may go through cycles of rupture and repair that are part of the process and can contribute to the strength of the relationship.

Tips

a) Mimic the child's vocalisations and actions if you think it will help you connect with him or her (do not be afraid to try).

b) The S-BRATA positions the therapist as an attachment figure; therefore, emulate behaviors that a mother would enact with her child.

c) Pay attention to your own bodily and emotional responses as they may be reflective of how the child is feeling.

d) Adjust body position, language and tone of voice to maintain safety and manage behaviors.

e) Be playful and go with the flow.

References

Benjamin, J. (1988). *The bonds of love.* New York, NY: Pantheon Book.

Csikszentmihalyi, M. (1990). *Flow: The psychology of optimal experience.* New York, NY: Harper Collins.

Evans, K., & Dubowski, J. (2001). *Art therapy with children on the autistic spectrum.* London, England: Jessica Kingsley.

Gallese, V. (2005). Embodied simulation: From neurons to phenomenal experience. *Phenomenology and Cognitive Sciences*, 4(1), 23–48. doi:10.1007/s11097-005-4737-z.

Henley, R. D. (2018). *Creative response activities for children on the spectrum*. New York, NY: Routledge.

Kossak, M. S. (2009). Therapeutic attunement: A transpersonal view of expressive arts therapy. *The Arts in Psychotherapy*, 36, 13–18. https://doi.org/10.1016/j.aip.2008.09.003.

Kossak, M. S. (2015). *Attunement in expressive arts therapy*. Illinois, USA: Charles Thomas Publishers.

Merleau-Ponty, M. (1962). *Phenomenology of perception* (Smith, C., trans.). London: Routledge & Keegan Paul.

Oberman, M. L., Pineda, A. J., & Ramachandaran, S. V. (2007) The human mirror neuron system: A link between action observation and social skills. *Social Cognitive and Affective Neuroscience*, 2(1), 62–66. doi:10.1093/scan/ns1022.

Stern, D. N. (1977). *The first relationship: Infant and mother*. Cambridge, MA: Harvard University Press.

Thaut, M., Kenyon, G., Schauer, M., & McIntosh, G. (1999). The connection between rhythmicity and brain function. *Engineering in Medicine and Biology Magazine*, 18(2), 101–108.

Warren, E. J., Sauter, A. D., Eisner, F., Wiland, J., Dresner, A. M., Wise, S. R., et al. (2006). Positive emotions preferentially engage an auditory-motor "mirror" system. *Journal of Neuroscience*, 26(50), 13067–13075. doi:10.1523/JNEUROSCI.3907-06.2006.

Wright, K. (2009). *Mirroring and attunement: Self-realization in psychoanalysis and art*. New York, NY: Routledge.

8 Art Materials as Entry Point of Engagement

Unlike other therapeutic interventions, art therapists have the unique advantage of access to a large variety of art materials and a deep understanding of their nature. The more traditional materials are the ones that most people are familiar with such as pencils, paints, crayons, clay, charcoal and so on; however, art can be made with virtually any material that evokes a creative response. Therefore, non-traditional materials like goop/slime or shaving foam may also be considered art materials due to their ability to engage the sensory, kinesthetic, affective and perceptual aspects of human expression in a creative way. The most obvious function of art materials is their capacity to produce images from application to a variety of surfaces, and in the case of malleable materials to make sculptures, shapes and forms, but the lesser known characteristic is their ability to induce and modulate affect, trigger memories and evoke emotional, symbolic and cognitive responses.

Through my sessions with Teo, Raj and Alex, I discovered that art materials were almost always the entry point of engagement with all three boys. I used the lure of art materials to motivate the boys into engaging with me, and once I had their attention, I could then focus on regulating them concurrent to the attachment work. I will illustrate my point through the case vignettes shared subsequently, but before that I have provided a summary of some of the traditional and non-traditional art materials and what I have learned from using them to make art myself and with my clients with and without ASD.

Traditional Art Materials

Paint

Paint is known for its emotive qualities due to its fluid nature and ability to tap into deep-seated emotional content. Malchiodi (2002) described it as having "a unique personality: it can be stimulating because of the color and brushstrokes, and at the same time hypnotic and almost sedating because of its fluidity" (p. 59). Paint is available in different formulations such as tempera, water colors, acrylics and oils. Water-based paints can be hard to control as opposed to oil-based ones that can be layered, influencing the level of affect. However, water-based paints are easier to wipe clean and wash out of clothes, an important consideration when working with children.

Paint is stored in tubes, bottles, jars and pans and can be applied with hands, a large variety of brushes, knives, sponges and any other material that can be dipped into it and applied to a surface. I keep paint in plastic squeeze bottles for pouring directly onto the paper because their nozzles can be cut to control the amount of paint dispensed. This is especially helpful with children who are likely to pour out large amounts of paint from wide mouthed containers, such as Alex who had a tendency to dysregulate with the material.

Paint can also be mixed with other materials to create a variety of textures. I have used different combinations of flour, paint, water, gravel and sand to be spread on an assortment of papers for tactile input. It is always a good idea to have plenty of paper towels and wet wipes around when using paint with children like Alex who spread it all over his face when hyper-aroused.

Paint may need to be used sparingly with children who tend to dysregulate easily. On the other hand, paint can be used to motivate and rouse passive children. It is an excellent medium to use when practicing self-regulation as it can be alternated with clay to induce and modulate affect consecutively as discussed in the section on sensory regulation.

Clay

Clay is primarily a "physical and kinesthetic" material that is "moist and amenable to being freely shaped" (McNiff, 1998, p. 29). Potter's clay is inherently earthy and is known for its ability to ground or contain affect. It is made from a mixture of earth and water and is used to make ceramics and sculptures. Self-hardening clay, also known as paper clay, is similar to potter's clay but does not require firing and may be painted on soon after drying. While potter's clay and paper clay are my personal favorites, I find that managing their consistency can get tricky for children and the interaction can end up being fairly messy, which may lead to regression. "Clay is a good medium for coming to know visceral experience. Strong, instinctual experiences lend themselves to expression in this simple material, which requires no tools but can be shaped directly with the pressure of your hands. If you wish to contact your gut, clay, which is slippery and dark and evokes dirt or even excrement, provides swift passage" (Allen, 1995, p. 703). While messy play may be the goal of therapy in some cases, I would recommend using synthetic clay for children who dysregulate easily and require grounding. Synthetic clay is available in many consistencies and colors and does not require adding water for pliability.

All types of clay may be pounded, kneaded, squeezed, rolled, coiled and moulded. Clay can be added to or taken away from to create forms and shapes. For children on the spectrum, clay can provide the proprioceptive and tactile input to the hyposensitive child who craves touch and pressure.

Conversely, a child who may be hyper-aroused and dysregulated can be pacified by the cool and compact nature of the material.

Pencils/Markers

Pencils and markers are relatively restrictive and rigid mediums that can be used for drawing, doodling, creating patterns and coloring. They are available in variety of colors, grips, thickness and degrees of hardness in the case of pencils. Pencils may be erased whereas markers are usually permanent, except for chalk or glass markers that can be wiped clean. I often begin a session by inviting children to draw large circles or patterns with glass markers using both hands on the mirrors in my studio. It is a great warm-up activity and ice breaker for dyads or groups of children. When used repetitively, pencils and markers can induce calm and lessen anxiety. Also, because both materials lend themselves to control, they are less likely to cause dysregulation as opposed to the more fluid mediums such as paint.

Crayons/Oil Pastels

Crayons and oil pastels are somewhat similar as in both produce bold permanent marks requiring more friction than pencils or markers. Crayons are mostly non-smudgeable whereas oil pastels can be blended in. I find using these materials after paint can induce calm in children, possibly due to the heavier proprioception that is necessary for application. One of my clients, a 14-year-old boy with autism and significant intellectual challenges, required heavy proprioception and had a tendency to break crayons while coloring with them. My initial reaction was to stop him from breaking the crayons but seeing that he enjoyed using them I put aside a box of thick crayons that he could break and color with. I felt that this activity satisfied his craving for proprioceptive input, following which he could work with other materials without destroying them.

Chalk Pastels

Chalk pastels are powdery and can be smudged and blended with fingers. They are fragile and have to be handled relatively carefully or they can break. The sensorial qualities of chalk pastels evokes a certain softness and calm awakening the haptic senses. I find myself drawn to chalk pastels when I am in a contemplative mood. Smudging them draws my deeper into reflection, often bringing up memories of childhood; however, with children on the spectrum I prefer using crayons that are more solid and resistive.

Collage

Any material that can be stuck onto a surface can be used for collage. Among other materials, peeled-off crayon labels, torn paper, pencil shavings, sand, tape, shells, beads, buttons and stickers are handy materials for collage.

Non-Traditional Art Materials

Materials such as shaving foam, goop, kinetic sand and plastic body parts are considered non-traditional in art therapy because they overlap with play therapy and expressive arts therapies. However, art therapists can make use of these for sensory artmaking or to include play in the sessions.

Shaving Foam

Shaving foam can be very handy and a great motivator for most children. The foam can be sprayed directly on the hands or practically any other surface. I use it often as a warm-up activity on the mirror-lined walls of my studio and encourage the use of both hands for cross-lateral stimulation. This works especially well to motivate shy clients to relax and open up. Foam can also be mixed with different colors and textures, like colored sand and glitter, to create interest. The entire routine with shaving foam is heavily sensorial and kinesthetic plus a lot of fun for most children. However, some children may be averse to dirtying their hands due to sensory or other issues, and foam like any other material must be used judiciously.

Goop/Slime

I have used both goop, which is thick and opaque, and slime, which is thinner and translucent. Both can be a major draw for most children and a good resource for joint sensory play and engagement. Following is a recipe that I have used successfully to make goop:

Mix ½ cup white glue with desired color of paint and pour in liquid starch (approximately ½ cup) in a thin stream while mixing the glue. The mixture will begin to thickens and form lumps. When it achieves the consistency of dough, pour it out of the bowl and knead with hands until pliable.

I use Elmer's® glue and a Elmer's® slime starter to make slime. The glue is available in a variety of colors including neon and with added glitter. There are plenty of recipes available on the internet for goop and slime, and I am sure new and improved versions are up for the taking.

The Lure of Art Materials

As mentioned above, art materials were an entry point of engagement between me and Teo, Raj and Alex. As Henley (2018) put it, "If one can find an intrinsic motivator, even the most severe child on the spectrum might overcome his shyness and interact or participate" (p. 51). Although Raj seemed to lose interest in art materials and artmaking as therapy progressed, the interaction I had with him was mostly through art materials. With Alex and Teo (see Figures 8.1 & 8.2), art materials continued to be a draw for more sustained engagement with me. Vignette 1 and 2 provide a glimpse into the role that art materials played in facilitating short but meaningful openings with Teo.

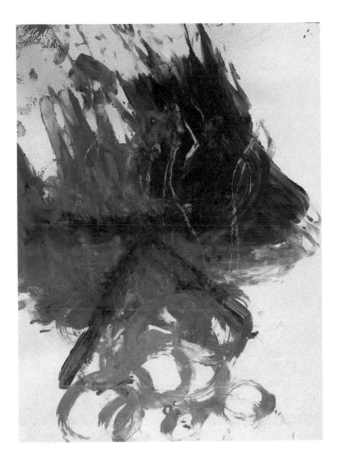

Figure 8.1 Teo: paint on paper

Vignette 1

Teo entered the waiting room crying. His mother shared that he was probably sleepy, and though he entered the studio willingly, he continued to
whine. Since Teo was obviously cranky, instead of approaching him actively,
I decided to step away from him and started playing with the brightly colored
goop I had prepared for the session. Standing on a plastic sheet, I began to
engage with the goop, which had turned out to be of a thinner consistency
than intended; however, that worked just as well because it allowed the
material to slip easily from my hands and flow onto the floor in long strands
that I attempted to catch. As I embellished my play with exaggerated "oohs"
and "aahs," Teo watched from a distance and gradually stopped whining.
Thenceforth, he walked up to me and took a piece of goop from my hand
before returning to his original spot in the room. He handled the goop for a

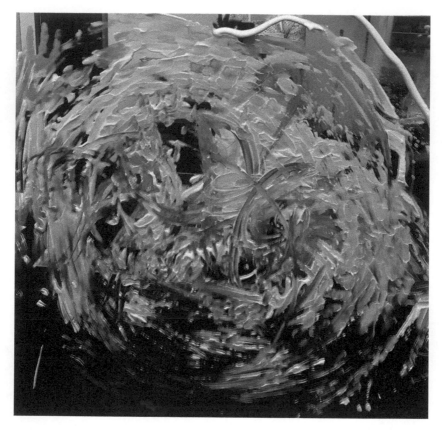

Figure 8.2 Teo: shaving foam on mirror

while and came back for more, moving it between his fingers before losing interest and abandoning it. Although my subsequent attempts to engage Teo with other art materials in the same session were met with fleeting interest, the goop proved to be a catalyst for Teo's despondent mood and provided some opportunity for proximity toward me.

Vignette 2

I began the session by throwing up a balloon to catch Teo's attention, but my performance did not seem to interest him. Leaving the balloon aside, I attempted to initiate a game of tag, but Teo looked at me in passing and continued to walk around the room preoccupied with his singing. Unfazed by his lack of response, I picked up a plastic tray and walked up to Teo holding a bottle of shaving foam. I squeezed out a blob of fluffy foam in close proximity to Teo's face so that there was no chance of him missing it. The shot of foam accompanied by the squirting sound caught Teo's interest and he grabbed the tray as I walked him back to a sheet of paper I had placed on the floor. I squeezed more foam onto the tray and Teo began to touch it and cover his hands with it. He seemed to enjoy the texture of the foam as he continued to wrap it around his hands and simultaneously his vocalisations became softer. Excited by Teo's involvement with the foam and eager to prolong it, I dropped a large drop of paint onto the paper and spread it with my finger. Teo, who was sitting beside the paper, noticed the splotch of color and touched it with his foam-covered hands. Spurred by Teo's attention, I covered my palms with paint and began to make hand prints on the paper and Teo turned to look at me. Hence, I added to the handprints with more colors in order to draw Teo further into the activity. Then Teo placed his foam-covered hand on the paper and I pressed it lightly to produce a print, exclaiming as his hand left its mark on the paper. It seemed that the process rather than the product was more appealing to Teo as he did not react to his handprint and began to spread the foam, now mixed with different colors of paint. Teo continued to rub the foam and paint mixture onto the paper and the tray lying next to it for a good 15 minutes before moving away. I was elated by Teo's sustained engagement with the foam and his response to my artmaking. He and I had been able to sit in close proximity longer than ever before.

Whereas Teo's reciprocal behaviors increased gradually with persistent coaxing with art materials, Alex from the start responded with enthusiasm to artmaking. Nevertheless, there were a couple of sessions where Alex was defiant and disruptive, and it was through art materials that I was able to redirect his behavior. For instance, during one session when it was time for Alex to go home, he ran and hid under the table, refusing to come out. After many minutes of cajoling him to come out, I grabbed some markers and began to draw on the mirror, offering Alex to join me by rolling a marker in his direction. Unable to resist, Alex slowly came out from under the table and began to draw alongside me before transitioning into goodbyes and heading home.

Lack of Motivation

Teo, Raj and Alex each reacted to art materials in a unique fashion. Teo's curiosity and engagement with the materials grew with the sessions and Alex's interest was consistent, whereas Raj's seemed to wane towards the end. From sessions one to nine, Raj intermittently engaged in sensory artmaking with shaving foam, sand, glitter, paint and glue. A few times he scribbled with crayons and even showed preference for certain colors; however, from session nine onward, there was a spike in Raj's stimming behaviors and he had a couple of big meltdowns. In these sessions where he showed very little interest in artmaking, I struggled with Raj's lack of response and felt lost and frustrated with no option but to sit through what seemed like rejection.

The vignette below describes one of the sessions where Raj showed considerable anger and was very upset. Art materials or perhaps the way I used them were not sufficient to regulate or motivate him. In the section under rupture and repair, I have explained how a break in attunement is part of the attachment process, and perhaps in session nine onward, Raj's and my relationship was going through such a period. Unfortunately, I did not have enough sessions left to work through the rupture with Raj due to the constraints of the study.

Vignette 3

Raj appeared to be excited and slightly aroused before the session. It was our second-last meeting and banking on the appeal of paint, sand and glue activity that he had enjoyed in an earlier session, I poured some paint on paper urging him to make handprints. Raj reacted by spreading paint with his hands instead of printing on the paper. I sensed his reluctance and lack of joy in the endeavor and, taking that as a cue, I should have backed off rather than encourage him to continue. Whether it was the tone of the session that I had set or something else entirely, Raj flew into a rage while I poured paint on his hand and began to scratch my arms. I was caught completely off guard as I had never seen him so angry before. I quickly got hold of shaving foam in order to divert Raj's attention and for a brief moment I thought I had succeeded before the tantrum resurfaced and Raj threw a container of pencils on the floor and broke into tears. Somewhat panicked, I grabbed hold of a pack of emotion cards that illustrated feelings like anger and sadness hoping that Raj would point to one (although, in retrospect even if he had, I am not sure how I would have carried the communication further considering his difficulty with language), but Raj continued to fret. Stumped by the intensity of Raj's tantrum and the lack of ideas, I backed off completely and sat in one part of the room and waited for Raj's rage to pass. Raj calmed down as I slowly began to clear the art materials and sang the goodbye song signalling the end of the session. Post-session discussion with Raj's mother revealed that he had been behaving similarly at home for the past week. His mother shared that she believed Raj may have been experiencing headaches that were responsible for his outbursts.

Sessions 9–12 with Raj, during which he appeared reluctant to engage with art materials and behaved aggressively at times, left me feeling that perhaps art materials were not always sufficient motivation for all children. Undoubtedly, they were an entry point of engagement between Raj and me, and there were times when we made art together, but I cannot be sure whether it was out of compulsion to respond to directives or the activity itself that afforded him pleasure. Perhaps if I had had the opportunity to work through the deadlock that I had reached with Raj, I would have found my answers.

Conclusion

The therapist can choose from a large variety of materials that when used judiciously provide opportunities for reciprocity and sustained relational activity. Art materials can be the entry point for engagement for children who lack motivation for communication and may also be used to detract from unwanted behaviors, especially if a child has a favorite material that can be used as an incentive. Art materials may not hold a strong enough appeal for some children and the therapist may have to improvise or include other expressive modalities to engage the child.

Tips

1) Use a large plastic sheet to protect the floor as it is easy to wipe clean.
2) Do not clutter the surface with too many art materials.
3) Always keep plenty of paper at hand in case more than a few sheets are required in quick succession.
4) Squeeze bottles for paints are a good way of controlling the amount of paint poured out, as are palettes with small indents.
5) Use paints that are easily washable.
6) For children with a tendency to put things in the mouth, it is necessary to use non-toxic art materials such as edible play dough and chemical-free paints.
7) Have kitchen paper roll and wet wipes handy at all times.
8) Keep toys such as balls, plastic dinner sets, small figures made from wood or plastic and musical instruments like shakers and drums. A selection of fidget and stim toys is a good idea.
9) Be ready to improvise if art materials are not a sufficient draw.

References

Allen, P. B. (1995). *Art is a way of knowing: A guide to self-knowledge and spiritual fulfilment through creativity* (Kindle Edition). Shambhala Publications.

Henley, R. D. (2018). *Creative response activities for children on the spectrum.* New York, NY: Routledge.

Malchiodi, A. C. (2002). *The soul's palette.* Boston, MA: Shambhala.

McNiff, S. (1998). *Trust the process.* Boston, MA: Shambhala.

9 Structure and Boundaries

Generally speaking, neurotypical individuals are well equipped to deal with everyday occurrences like shopping, eating out at a restaurant or going for a walk, barring ill health or extraordinary circumstances. However, for individuals with autism, sensory, relational and psychomotor variances can complicate the simplest of tasks. They may struggle to make sense of a constantly changing world that continuously exacts attention, selection, regulation and integration of input. A seemingly straightforward task like walking down the road that a neurotypical person may take for granted can present a navigational nightmare for an individual with ASD who may have challenges across multiple sensory domains. Similarly, a crowded classroom of children with limited space for each child, bursting with a cacophony of sounds and images, textures and forms, coupled with the expectation of performance could be a daunting prospect for an auditory sensitive, hyper-responsive child on the spectrum with a limited attention span. Nevertheless, output is necessary for survival whether it is to perform basic life skills or accomplish more complicated tasks. Since our environment is constantly changing and change is not necessarily linear, the outcome can be chaotic and the unpredictability alarming for individuals who are already battling an awry sensory system. In the words of Higashida (2007), "There are times when I can't do what I want to, or what I have to. It doesn't mean I don't want to do it. I just can't get it all together, somehow. Even performing one straightforward task, I can't get started as smoothly as you can…. There are times when I can't act, even though I really badly want to. This is when my body is beyond my control" (p. 40).

Unsurprisingly, then, people on the spectrum respond well to structure since it lends order, simplifies tasks and is predictable. It is a well-known fact that individuals with autism do very well in jobs that are highly structured and in fact are sought after by employers for their diligence and precision. Just as structure is dependable, boundaries provide containment and consistency, and the combination of both structure and boundaries translates into a sense of safety. Consequently, most behavioral interventions for children with ASD such as TEACCH and ABA are designed to accommodate the need for consistency, clarity and repetition. Reality, however, is not as dependable or accommodating and may be extremely anxiety provoking for children with autism; hence, helping children generalise their skills from the therapy room to their environment is one of the goals of the aforementioned behavioral interventions. This is done by scaffolding the child through exposure and practice to real-life situations in manageable doses and reinforcing adaptation skills and coping mechanisms.

Directive Versus Non-Directive Approaches in Art Therapy

Art therapy is not known to be a highly structured intervention in the sense of the behavioral approaches specific for ASD. That is not to say that there is a lack of organisation or predictability within the sessions, but largely therapists work in the present moment and tend to follow the lead of their clients. Art therapists may use directive or non-directive approaches or a mix of both depending upon their inclination and judgment. A non-directive approach is loosely structured, where the client determines the focus of the session while the therapist holds the space and facilitates reflection and re-solution where possible. Each session is built upon the previous one steered by the therapist's ongoing assessment of his or her client.

Conversely, where a directive approach is employed, the therapist may have a predetermined plan and goals for the session that are achieved through specific instructions pertaining to the topic or use of art material. Even so, within the framework of the directive, the client has the freedom to express him- or herself freely. There is no coercion to make art or to adhere to rigid boundaries.

The relatively unstructured nature of art therapy can present a challenge when working with children with autism who are used to the predictability of behavioral interventions that the majority are undergoing. I am speaking from my experience in Singapore where most of the children with ASD I have worked with so far are predominantly involved in behavior-focused therapies. In my work with children with autism, prior to my study with Teo, Raj and Alex, I was inclined to employ a mix of directive and non-directive approaches that were loosely structured, in that I would plan activities that I could use to achieve a specific goal but was not necessarily bound by them. I tended to follow the lead of the children and allowed them to dictate the amount of structure and boundaries that were necessary for them, and I followed the same principle with Teo, Raj and Alex. Some interventions like TEACCH modify the environment to facilitate orderliness; however, I deliberately resisted creating a highly structured environment within my studio in favor of a more natural one that would simulate a homey environment conducive to attachment work. Although the S-BRATA is not a highly structured approach, my sessions with Teo, Raj and Alex presented me with the opportunity of incorporating some degree of structure and boundaries that were necessary to manage certain behaviors and regulation issues.

The work done by art therapists Aach-Feldman and Kunkle-Miller (2016) provides some insight into how the therapist may progress from non-directive work with traditional and pre-art material to structured work with traditional or pre-art material depending on the developmental stage of the child. Based on their experience with children on the spectrum, Gabriels and Gaffey (2012) suggested the use of visual schedules, picture-word instructions and breaking down tasks into multiple steps to provide structure and consistency. The vignettes below are illustrative of my experience with the theme of structure and boundaries.

Boundaries

As mentioned before, Alex had a tendency toward hyper-arousal with paint, but paint was his favorite art material as well, and unsurprisingly, he would ask for it in each session. Alex used paint primarily for sensory exploration and not so much for creating images. He enjoyed pouring out the paint, often excessively, then chose either rollers or brushes to apply it on paper before planting his hands onto wet paint and smearing his face with it. Subsequently, Alex did not enjoy the process of having me wipe the paint off his face, and once or twice it almost went into his eyes. Therefore, I informed Alex that paint on the face was off limits, but he was not compliant, indicating the need for firmer boundaries. Below I describe how I learned to adjust boundaries with Alex over successive sessions, resulting in some degree of success.

Vignette 1

In this particular session, when Alex asked for paint, I told him before he could start using it that I did not want him to put it on his face. I laid out the a palette with small indents and indicated that Alex could fill up the material up to the rim of the indents. Alex was given paint in squeeze bottles that were half filled with thick paint that would not spill out easily. My instructions urging constraint seemed to have had an impact as Alex only poured enough paint to fill the indents on the palette, whereas in previous sessions he would swiftly grab the bottles of paint and squeeze out large amounts of it before I could intervene. Once the paint had been poured into the palette, Alex began stamping the paint on paper with sponges and from there the stamping moved onto his arms and eventually to his face. Apparently, my attempt at setting boundaries had only succeeded up to the pouring of the paint and not to its application on Alex's face.

In the following session, when Alex asked for paint again, I decided to be more explicit with communicating the limits that he was expected to comply with. Perhaps a verbal prompt had been insufficient and added to it a visual one would be more emphatic. Therefore, I drew a face with paint laden hands and put a big cross on it verbalising that Alex was not allowed to smear his face. I placed the drawing in front of Alex so that he could see it at all times and we shook hands on it! Alex wanted to do roller printing and a few times he attempted to squirt out excessive paint from the squeeze bottles, but I was quick to redirect him by tipping the back end of the bottle in his hand and directing his gaze to the visual prompt. Alex continued to make marks with the roller on paper (see Figure 9.1), and I praised him profusely for his good work and for maintaining boundaries. At last, Alex had refrained from putting paint on his face and I happily moved him onto the next activity.

Alex continued to push boundaries in the following sessions, one way or another. If it wasn't covering his face with paint, it would be refusal to leave the room after the session was over or conversely to enter it in the first place. Whether his behaviors stemmed from difficulty with transitions, challenges with self-regulation or plain rigidity, it became clear to me that Alex required clear and consistent boundaries.

I agree with Martin that "[c]hildren in general usually stay on task better with instruction and incentives, and for children experiencing symptoms that interfere with attention span and appropriate art play, it is imperative to create these conditions" (Martin, 2009, p. 113). Especially with Alex, who had good receptive and expressive language, clear instruction and firm boundaries were the way to go. But with children where functional language is absent, as was with Teo, there may not be the need for strict boundaries since Teo was not at the level of engagement or reciprocity where I was required to set them. The primary focus in Teo's case was motivating him to come out of his shell to begin to interact with his environment; hence, Teo's case, as compared to Alex's, required a contrasting approach when it came to imposing boundaries.

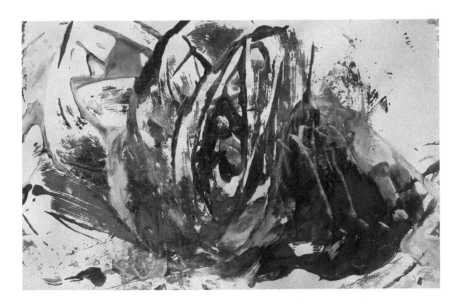

Figure 9.1 Alex: painting with rollers

Structure

Structuring a session for a child such as Alex, who was responsive and could follow instructions, was far easier than doing so for Teo and Raj, who were unresponsive and resistant, respectively. My initial stance with all three boys was to follow their lead and allow their progression to guide my approach. Thus, in Alex's case, just as his behaviors dictated the need for boundaries, his sessions organically developed a structure. For instance, cognizant of Alex's short attention span, I always had a line-up of art materials and activities that I could use in the session in quick succession to sustain interest. As the sessions proceeded, I was able to pre-empt Alex's preference for a particular material or activity, and that resulted in a routine in which, for example, he would start with paint, followed by sand play or stamping and pasting with intermittent breaks. In a sense, there was an element of predictability in the sessions with Alex that was missing from Teo and Raj's sessions. With Teo, my goal was to foster an innate desire in him to connect, and for that to happen, the sessions were loosely structured based on his motivation and initiative. As for Raj, who was able to respond to directives but was harder to motivate with art materials than Teo, I struggled between wanting to impose a structure but not really knowing how to. My challenge was that the art materials nor any activity that I had tried to introduce into the sessions was motivating enough to sustain Raj's attention. Perhaps Raj would have benefited with a highly structured approach that I was not able to provide. The following vignettes illustrate the combination of structure and boundaries through two successive sessions with Alex.

Vignette 2

Alex refused to leave his mother and enter the art therapy room. I attempted to tempt him with the foam face cut-outs, a material he had not worked with before, hoping that it would pique his interest. Drawn by curiosity, Alex followed me into the room but his body language but I sensed his reluctance, almost as if he had forced himself to come in. Nevertheless, I modeled for him how to draw features on the foam cut outs and Alex followed suit but that was the end of his artmaking for this session. Henceforth, his behavior in the session escalated into complete defiance and testing my boundaries. Alex threw the foam cut outs into the trash bin, his as well as mine, and proceeded to jumble the wool that I had taken out to make hair for the faces. He moved away from me so that I could not stop him from unravelling the ball of wool and snipping it with scissors. Afraid that he may injure himself with the scissors in this hyper-aroused state, I calmly asked him to hand them over but Alex ran out of the room into the waiting room to his mother. By now Alex was throwing a full blown tantrum and was completely unreceptive to my or his mother's attempts to calm him down. I decided that it was best to shorten the session and send Alex home with the message that this kind of behavior was unacceptable. When Alex realised that he was being taken home and that I had ended the session, his tantrum escalated further and he refused to leave, insisting that he wanted to re-enter the studio. However, Alex was unable to calm down, and I decided to stand my ground and sent him home.

In the following session, Alex was again resistant to come in. Not wanting to coerce him, I indicated that he was free to go home. However, Alex once again refused to do that as well, repeating the pattern of the previous session. Finally, he came into the room and I was able to catch his attention with the magic paper that was new to him. Alex scratched the magic paper with a wooden pen to reveal a multicolored drawing underneath, and it kept him busy for a while. I had already planned the next activity in my head, cognizant of Alex's short attention span, and directed him to painting. A planned succession of activities lent some structure to the sessions with Alex as it did not allow too much free time, which tended to dysregulate him. Also, moving from one task to another provided a degree of predictability and containment, although that did not necessarily ensure a smooth session. Subsequently, Alex was able to make three artworks with paint, sand and glue. I controlled the amount of paint by tipping the squeeze as he poured the material out of them and insisting that I pour the glue while he poured out the sand. Alex finally seemed to be enjoying the session, yet I sensed an underlying tension in him reflected in his stiff body posture and quick movements. By now I had the third activity in place, which consisted of play dough and the comic body parts that Alex had responded to well in the past. A malleable material like clay or play dough compensated well for the freedom of paint and kept Alex grounded. However, unpredictability is part of the challenge of working with children on the spectrum, and Alex erupted into disorderly behavior after the play dough activity. He ran to the waiting room where his mother was not present to pick him up and spilled water from the water dispenser onto the floor. Next, Alex started banging on the door and throwing things around the room until his mother returned and told him to go home, but he refused to budge and insisted that he wanted to go back into the studio. I stood in front of the art therapy room, with a clear message that re-entry was not possible.

In subsequent sessions, Alex's behavior calmed down considerably. It is possible he had internalised the boundaries that I had set for him in terms of acceptable and unacceptable behaviors. I continued to maintain the loose structure and firm boundaries through the remaining sessions with Alex.

Conclusion

Children on the spectrum generally respond well to structure. A directive approach lends itself to structure but may be combined with a non-directive one, especially within the framework of the S-BRATA in which the goal is not to teach skills but to establish an attachment with the child. A rigid structure may compromise the therapist's ability to emulate attachment behaviors in a naturalistic environment. Having said that, some degree of structure and/or boundaries may be necessary for children with autism as is the case with most typical children.

Tips

- Let the child guide how much structure and boundary are necessary, experiment with incremental increase and adjust accordingly.
- Be consistent with the boundaries and stand your ground, especially when managing disruptive behaviors.
- Impulsive behaviors and erratic responses can catch the therapist off guard, but unpredictability is inherent in working with children with ASD.

References

Aach-Feldman, S., & Kunkle-Miller, C. (2016). Developmental art therapy. In Rubin, A. R. (Ed.), *Approaches to art therapy* (pp. 435–451). New York, NY: Routledge.

Gabriels, L. R., & Gaffey, J. L. (2012). Art therapy with children on the autism spectrum. In Malchiodi, A. C. (Ed.), *Handbook of art therapy* (2nd ed., pp. 205–221). New York, NY: The Guilford Press.

Higashida, N. (2007). *The reason I jump*. New York, NY: Random House.

Martin, N. (2009). *Art as an early intervention tool for children with autism*. London, UK: Jessica Kingsley.

10 Flexibility

The landscape of the profession of art therapy has changed dramatically from its inception in psychoanalysis to a vastly broader discipline that espouses diverse orientations from psychodynamic psychology to humanistic, cognitive, systemic, neuroscience and developmental, among others. Art therapy practice has grown beyond the confines of a therapy room to reach a wider community through the community art studio, embracing social action in times of natural disasters and calamities across the world. Therapists themselves have evolved from being the experts in the field to co-creators and collaborators, adopting the social constructionist view of not knowing and trusting the individuals' capacity to take charge of their lives. This decidedly postmodern stance, which is rooted in humanistic approaches, positions the client as a partner, challenging the hierarchical order of the client-therapist relationship (Rubin, 2016). This dynamism within art therapy research and practice is reflected in the distinct orientations that contemporary art therapists have adopted and developed in the last couple of decades. In her book *Approaches to Art Therapy*, Judith Aron Rubin described art therapy as a *hybrid* discipline with *"art as the core."* Highlighting the theoretical roots of art therapy in psychology and psychiatry, she noted how profession has evolved to include a range of expressive modalities reflected in the practice of current art therapists such as Henley and Mcniff, among others. For instance, Henley illustrated an integrated arts therapy approach where he used a combination of "art, photography, poetry and bibliotherapy" as a teacher/ therapist to provide therapeutic support to teenagers in a school setting (Henley, 2016, p. 466). Similarly, iterating the benefits of incorporating a hybrid stance, McNiff (2016) demonstrated how the different art forms complement and enhance each other, such as making art to the beat of percussive instruments and incorporating movement and rhythm while painting. On the other hand, Aach-Feldman and Kunkle-Miller (2016) illustrated an entirely separate methodology by employing a developmental art therapy approach with children, based on psychoanalytic, cognitive and developmental theories. Their stance is focused on incorporating sensory exploration with art materials with the inclusion of songs and play. According to Wadeson (2016), individuality of therapeutic style is inevitable since "the selfhood of each therapist is unique, each clinician's creative work in this realm will bear the imprimatur of that self, with all its life experience influencing each moment of the therapeutic relationship (p. 479).

The gradual broadening of the scope of art therapy as art therapists grow more secure with their identity as artists and therapists (Rubin, 2016) can nevertheless lead to concerns about a confused eclecticism (McNiff, 2016), especially for those who are trained in one specific modality such as art, drama or music. I faced this dilemma early on in my career where I was impelled to adopt a developmental approach from a decidedly psychody-namic one and was thrust into unknown territory that almost felt like a betrayal of my beliefs about what art therapy was supposed to be. As I practiced, I learned, adapted and was able to let go of rigid preconceptions and limiting determinisms that can stymie creativity and reflexive practice. Therefore, during the formulation of the S-BRATA, cognizant of my lim-itations in the broader arts therapies, I was willing to push the boundaries of my own comfort zone to meet the varied needs of Teo, Raj and Alex. While my primary focus was the multisensory use of art materials and artmaking for sensory regulation and attachment formation, I included elements of play and music in the sessions to motivate the boys and to encourage reciprocal be-haviors. The need for flexibility across all the themes of the S-BRATA became increasingly apparent due to the complexity of the spectrum and the unpredictability of each child's response from one session to the other.

The Space as a Playground

My art therapy room was large enough (approximately 400 square feet) to accommodate two sets of tables and chairs, the bigger set for adolescents and adults and the smaller one suitable for children up to 10 years old. Besides these pieces of furniture, there was plenty of room for storage, a few cushions and a couple of large beanbags and yet there was a big space for floor-based activities in the center. I view my studio as the parallel of a children's playground where art materials, musical instruments and toys are replacements for swings and slides. Just as a child is free to explore the nooks and crannies of a playground and enjoy the paraphernalia, an art therapy room should be a place of discovery and excitement. As Winnicott (1971) stated, "It is in playing and only in playing that the individual child or adult is able to be creative and to use the whole personality, and it is only in being creative that the individual discovers the self" (p. 72–73). Hence, all parts of the studio can be a place for engaging with art materials or artmaking, whether it is on tables or chairs, lying down on the floor, coloring or smearing shaving foam on the walls (in my case, the mirror-lined walls of my room), as long as the child's safety is not compromised.

I would like to believe that I was able to emulate the environment of a playground within my art therapy room for Teo, Raj and Alex. They had complete freedom to run around the room and make art on whichever surface they felt comfortable. I spread large plastic sheets to protect the floor from damage and had to remove the upholstered chairs after they were smothered in paint by Teo's handprints. There were times after a session with Teo where I had to spend a good half hour cleaning the room since his lack of body awareness meant that there was paint smeared on the walls and the furniture as well as play dough stuck onto the floor where he had walked over it. Admittedly, at times when Teo walked around the room with foam- and paint-laden hands that would inevitably end up on my wall or cushions, I would catch myself grimacing. However, my awareness of his limitations and the fact that I wanted him to own the space motivated me to be as flexible as I could with the use of the room. When working with pre-art materials such as sand, foam, goop, etc., it may be difficult to restrict engagement on one particular surface, especially if the child is inclined to seek movement and may be hyper-aroused. I discovered I was less stressed and my body language more relaxed when I got comfortable with the children using the art materials freely without fear of marking my furniture with paint or plastering it with foam. Following is an example of a session where Raj made use of different surfaces in the room and I was happy to follow his lead. We moved from the floor to the table and then back to the floor, engaging with a variety of art material. I even played the xylophone to end the session and it was not the first time that I wished I had proficiency in playing a musical instrument.

Vignette 1

I sat next to the art materials on the floor and called Raj to join me. He approached me and gave me a hug around my back. I felt that he was comfortable and familiar. I began to make art while Raj picked up the brush he usually used for stimming and held it close to his chin, feeling the bristles. I prompted him to join me in my artmaking and but after making a few marks on paper, Raj seemed to tire of it. He moved toward the large table and I followed him. After he climbed onto the chair, I pushed a box of crayons toward him. Raj began digging his nails into the crayons and then marked his arm with them. I mirrored his action by doing the same with his other arm. Next Raj moved back to the floor and I followed him. Once again I attempted to engage Raj pouring the paint on the paper, hoping it would motivate him to dip his fingers or make brush marks. Raj touched the paint with fingers and I modeled finger painting for him, wanting him to follow my lead, but Raj grabbed the piece of paper that lay between us and began to tear it up accompanied by loud vocalisations. I tried to redirect his behavior by illustrating how to crush the paper and quickly grabbed white glue, sand and buttons to expand the activity. I estimated that glue and sand would provide Raj a stronger sensory experience and indeed, he seemed to enjoy the texture of glue and sand mixed together (see Figure 10.1). While I tried to direct the application of the media onto the paper, Raj was keen to just feel them. The session ended playing me playing the xylophone in the last 10 minutes, giving Raj time to transition into saying goodbye.

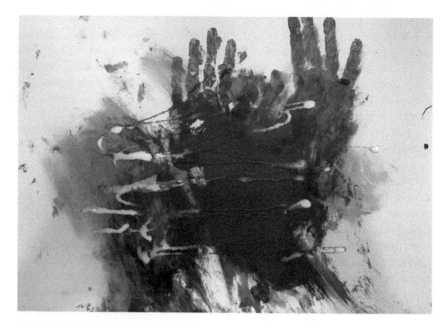

Figure 10.1 Raj: paint, sand and glue

The vignette below is an illustration of how I moved from one activity to another to motivate Teo to engage with me. I used a variety of art materials and surfaces to catch Teo's attention, eventually resorting to holding back due to lack of response from him.

Vignette 2

Teo was cranky and crying when he entered the waiting room. His mother said he was probably sleepy; however, he entered the studio without resistance as if on cue. I moved to the center of the room where I had placed the plastic sheet on the floor and began to engage with the goop that I had prepared for the session. I manipulated the soft and malleable material, stretching it with my hands in exaggerated movements to pique Teo's interest. He watched me from his end of the room and after a few minutes came up to me and took a piece of goop from my hand before moving away. The goop could not hold his interest for long, and he did not ask for more. Although Teo had stopped crying once he entered the room, his energy was low and pulled me down with it. Giving up on the goop, I moved on to roller painting on a large sheet of paper, adding glue and sand to the paint to create texture, hoping that Teo, who sought tactile input, would enjoy the consistency of the mixture. However, Teo did not budge, and I once again had to abandon my position and move on to another activity, wishing for something to work. Shaving foam had motivated Teo to engage in earlier sessions, so grabbing the can of foam I went up to the mirror and squeezed out blobs of foam to spread in large circles with my hand. Teo approached the mirror and finally went for the foam and covered his hands with it, but he was not keen to apply it to the mirror. Rather, he went over to the sofas in the corner of the room and rubbed his foam-laden hands all over the upholstery. Teo's lack of awareness of the environment and his sense of proprioception or his body in space instigated acts that were not really intentional but rather were driven by his sensory needs. Thus, after wiping his hands over the sofas, Teo walked over the roller painting on the floor, oblivious to the marks his paint covered shoes were making. Somewhat disappointed by Teo's lack of response, I spent the rest of the session making art by myself in one part of the room deciding to hold back further engagement till Teo was ready.

Toys, Musical Instruments and More

I have a small collection of basic play therapy toys such as fairy tale figurines, superheroes, soldiers, fantastical creatures, a castle, a bridge, a well and a trunk that I keep in two trays; a plastic jar that contains cartoon body parts that can be stuck on shapes made with clay or play dough (see Figure 10.2); a small plastic tea set complete with plates and cutlery and a container of pretend food. I keep a lookout for interesting balls in various sizes, colors, interesting textures, firmness and bounce. It is always a good idea to have a large soft ball that is easy to catch and safe to throw if there is a chance of misjudgment. Some squish balls that can be squeezed are good stress busters and can also work as stim objects for tactile and proprioceptive input. Similarly, rubber toys that can be tugged and stretched may catch the fancy of some children like Alex, who had a special liking for a green caterpillar that he liked to hold onto. I also keep some musical instruments such as drums, shakers and a xylophone that can come in handy as distractions, motivators or for opening and closing rituals. My inflatable sand tray that came with a set of plastic molds, sand tool and kinetic sand is a great motivator for some children who enjoy building with the molds and improvising activities with the sand. With Teo, Raj and Alex, I made use of some of the material mentioned above as and when I felt the need to motivate them. Artmaking, engaging with toys and musical instruments would sometimes be interspersed with a game of hide and seek with Alex, attempts to play catch with Teo and beating the drums for Raj. Following are two examples where I used a combination of play and artmaking with Alex to achieve the dual purpose of sensory regulation and relational artmaking.

Vignette 3

Five minutes into session, Alex went up to the tray of toys. He rummaged through it before the tea set lying next to it caught his interest. Allowing

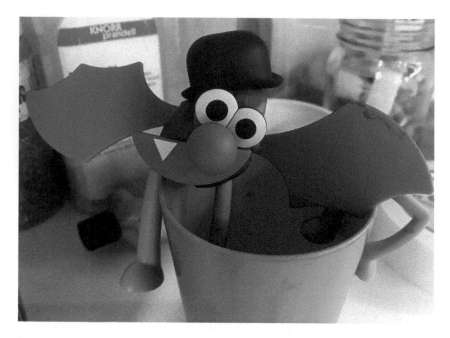

Figure 10.2 Alex: clay with plastic body parts

Alex some time to explore the tea set, I approached him with a piece of play dough to improvise play between us. I helped Alex carry the tea set back to the table where we laid it down to make pretend food for each other with the play dough, and he and I shared the food building a conversation around it. Alex appeared to enjoy the activity immensely and asked multiple times if I wanted more coffee so that he could refill my cup. I gladly drank multiple cups of coffee, making Alex's favorite foods and feeding him in the tiny plates. Our play with the tea set lasted approximately 10 minutes, which was a fair long of time for Alex to stay with one activity since he had a short attention span. I took cue from Alex's interest in the moment, in this case a toy, to devise a way to pair the activity with art material to target the sensory work that I wanted to do with him. The manipulation of the play dough kept Alex grounded while the pretend play turned into an enjoyable bonding experience through mutual nurturance.

Another play-based activity that Alex thoroughly enjoyed was a sand tray activity where he and I took turns to bury figurines of superheroes and fairy tale creatures under a mountain of kinetic sand and then excavate them. The burier would secretly bury the toys under the mound of sand while the excavator had to close his or her eyes and wait. Subsequently, the excavator would have to dig through the sand with hands or sand tools to unearth the buried figurines. For Alex, the process of discovery was filled with great anticipation and excitement that I augmented with animated gestures and dialogue. We were able to do multiple rounds of the burying and excavating routine, so much so that I would tire of it before Alex. However, this activity was ideal for the occasions where I needed to provide some grounding to Alex, especially after using a fluid medium such as paint that caused high arousal in him. It facilitated the practice of regulation while keeping Alex happily employed.

Conclusion

There is no place for rigidity in the S-BRATA. The theme of flexibility stresses adaptation, adjustment, improvisation and the setting aside of pre-conceived expectations or ideas that delimit relational activity with the child with autism. What it means is that though the framework has emerged from a primarily art therapy intervention, it allows for inclusion of play, music, drama, movement and other forms of creative expression.

Tips

a) Flexibility is the key to success.
b) Follow the lead of the child.
c) Build the session around the child's area of interest, be it toys, music or art.
d) Do not be afraid to push your boundaries and be open to new learning all the time.

References

Aach-Feldman, S., & Kunkle-Miller, C. (2016). Developmental art therapy. In Rubin, A. R. (Ed.), *Approaches to art therapy* (pp. 435–451). New York, NY: Routledge.

Henley, D. (2016). Lessons in the images. Developmental art therapy. In Rubin, A. R. (Ed.), *Approaches to art therapy* (pp. 452–467). New York, NY: Routledge.

McNiff, S. (2016). Pandora's gifts. Developmental art therapy. In Rubin, A. R. (Ed.), *Approaches to art therapy* (pp. 468–478). New York, NY: Routledge.

Rubin, J. A. R. (2016). Introduction. In Rubin, A. R. (Ed.), *Approaches to art therapy* (pp. 1–14). New York, NY: Routledge.

Wadeson, H. (2016). An eclectic approach to art therapy. In Rubin, A. R. (Ed.), *Approaches to art therapy* (pp. 479–492). New York, NY: Routledge.

Winnicott, D. W. (1971). *Playing and reality*. New York, NY: Basic Books.

11 Art Product Not the Focus

Children with autism struggle with symbolic thought and expression in varying degrees. Symbolism is an acquired ability that emerges from the cascading effect of developmental skills such as joint attention and shared affect that develop in the first year of an infant's life (Charman & Stone, 2006). Consequently, these fundamental building blocks of reciprocal communication and shared meanings culminate in receptive and expressive language. In turn, language, which is a complex synthesis of verbal and nonverbal communication, speech perception, comprehension, vocabulary development and so on, influences the advancement of symbolic thought. Earlier, under the topic of SID, I discussed how children on the spectrum have significant deficits in the apparatus of social-affective mechanisms such as eye gaze, preferential attention, intensity of eye contact and referential looking that directly affect the skill of joint attention, and, together with other developmental challenges such as cognitive ability and sensory issues, it is not surprising that the capacity to symbolise in children with autism is impacted. It is prudent, then, to assume that the development of symbolism in children with ASD would correspond to the severity of the presence of aforementioned deficits, meaning a child who has deep autism would have a much more diminished capacity for symbolic thought as opposed to a child who is not as deeply affected.

Teo's and Raj's expressions were indicative of a lack of capacity to symbolise, which was consistent with their considerable communication challenges. Alex, on the other hand, showed some development of symbolic thought where there was the emergence of an art product; however, it is safe to say that for all three boys, the artmaking was very much sensory based and may be considered pre-art in the case of Teo and Raj. However, that does not mean that their process of engaging with art materials for sensory gratification leading to occasional mark making was not imbued with meaning. According to Henley (2018), "children may manipulate sand, water, cotton balls and blocks, but these activities are akin to play rather than endowing the activity with symbolism. The first stage towards symbolization is that of 'making special'" (p. 78). Henley's use of the term *making special* resonates deeply with the kind of art that Teo, Raj and Alex made in the sessions, in that it may not have culminated in the abstract expression of higher-level thought processes but, nevertheless, it was meaningful to them within the scope of their developmental capacity. According to Morgan (1995), "any art form is one of many possible statements about some kind of human experience" (p. 3) and in the case of the aforementioned boys, it would not be wrong to say that their artmaking was indeed a sensory-based relational experience.

Below I describe Teo's, Raj's and Alex's artmaking using the ETC, Piaget's stages of development (Piaget, 1954) and Lowenfeld's (1947) stages of artistic development (see Tables 11.1 and 11.2) as points of reference for where the boys could be operating in terms of their expressive and developmental abilities.

Teo

Through the span of Teo's sessions with me, his artmaking primarily remained on the kinesthetic and sensory levels of the ETC. Though there was an interdependence of the two polarities in Teo, it appeared that he had a stronger pull toward the sensory end of the spectrum as a lot of his engagement with art materials was tactile based. According to Piaget's stages of

Piaget's Stages of Cognitive Development and their primary characteristics
The Sensorimotor stage (birth to 2 years)
<ul><li>Infants learn from movement, sensations and actions</li><li>There is emergence of object permanence and establishment of cause and effect</li><li>Children learn that they have a distinct identity from their environment</li><li>In the later part of the stage, representational thought may emerge</li></ul>
The Preoperational Stage (2-7 years)
<ul><li>Children use words and pictures to represent objects</li><li>There develop pretend play skills and language skills but struggle with logic and the idea of constancy</li><li>They struggle with seeing other people's perspective and are egocentric</li></ul>
The Concrete Operational Stage (7-11 years)
<ul><li>Children become much more adept at logic and perspective taking</li><li>While still very rigid, they realise that others may not share their thoughts and feel differently</li><li>They may struggle with abstract concepts</li></ul>
The Formal Operational Stage (12 + years)
<ul><li>There is emergence of abstract thought, theoretical reasoning and deductive logic</li><li>Teens develop the ability to think about abstract ideas and logic and plan for the future</li></ul>

Table 11.1 Piaget's Stages of Cognitive Development and their primary characteristics

---

The Scribbling Stage (2 years)

- The first scribbles are *disordered* or uncontrolled markings leading on to *longitudinal* or *circular* scribbles that are relatively controlled and more complex. The focus is on movement that lends pleasure through kinesthetic exploration. There is no intention to portray the visual world.

- An important milestone of this stage is called *naming* when the child begins to name the scribbles, progressing from motion to thinking in pictures. The child may tell a story about the scribble as the imagination develops.

The Pre-schematic Stage (4-6 years)

- At this stage the schema or visual idea of the human or animal forms emerges as represented by a circle for the head and two vertical lines as the legs. The drawing depicts the most significant aspects of the objects to the child. There is not much understanding of space and colour is used emotionally and unrealistically. Objects may be floating and placed haphazardly.

The Schematic Stage (7-9 years)

- The concept of space emerges and the use of the horizon and sky line in drawings illustrates the development of relationships between objects. Colours are depicted realistically. Objects may be drawn with exaggerated features, for example person is taller than the house, reflecting the child's focal point or feelings. X-ray drawings are common where the inside and the outside of the subject are shown.

Dawning Realism (9-11 years)

- This stage is marked by awareness of the lack of ability to draw objects realistically which leads to self-criticism and focus on details rather than the image as a whole. Perspective appears in drawings and shading may be used to create three dimensional effect. Space may be represented by over lapping and experimenting with size of subjects. Artwork may appear to be less spontaneous and rigid as compared to previous stages.
-

Pseudorealistic (11-13 years)

- The end result takes precedence over the process of artmaking. Two types of artistic styles may appear: visual and non-visual. The visual artist is focused on the logical interpretation of the object whereas the non-visual artist uses the artwork for emotional expression.

Table 11.2 Lowenfeld's Stages of Artistic Development

development, Teo's would be placed at the sensorimotor stage that corresponds to 0–2 years of age, in which children learn about the world mainly through sensory experiences (Piaget, 1954). This is consistent with Lowenfeld's scribble stage (2 years), where Teo's engagement with the art material was driven entirely by kinesthetic rather than visual pleasure.

Therefore, Teo's performance on the ETC is consonant with his developmental age according to Piaget and Lowenfeld's stages of artistic development. Aach-Feldman and Kunkle Miller's following quote describes Teo to the tee…according to the authors, "the normal sense of curiosity leading to investigating the world, as well as the pleasure from that exploration, are often lacking in the developmentally delayed client. Motivation of clients at this stage is a difficult task, one which must take-into-account the functioning level, interests and chronological issues" (Aach-Feldman & Kunkle Miller, 2016, p. 438). Hence, the art product in Teo's case was not even a consideration as it was his process of engaging with the art materials through which he was able to establish a meaningful relationship with me that was significant. I am inclined to believe that Teo's process was not without meaning as it facilitated his connection with the outside world and instigated a process of communication that has implications for the growth of social-affective mechanisms described earlier.

Raj

Similarly, Raj, much like Teo, also functioned at the kinesthetic and sensory levels of the ETC. The challenge with Raj was that he required as much kinesthetic engagement as the sensory and whereas I was able to provide him with the latter, perhaps I was not so successful in incorporating the former. Hence, although Raj remained more toward the sensory polarity of the ETC while artmaking, it is possible that had I been able to facilitate more movement through engagement with the art materials, there would have been a more effective balance between the kinesthetic and sensory ends of the continuum. Thus Raj, like Teo, would qualify for Piaget's sensorimotor stage of development and Lowenfeld's scribble stage. However, in one session, Raj showed some indication of emergence to the Piaget's pre-operational stage (2–7 years of age) where he pointed to a stick figure I had made and named it "mama." According to Lowenfeld, Raj's ability to associate the visual idea with a human form points to a leap to the pre-schematic stage of artistic development (4–6 years). This corresponds with Piaget's pre-operational stage, which is signified by the beginning of symbolic thought and use of words and pictures to represent objects. Nevertheless, Raj's complete lack of interest in the marks he made rendered the art product irrelevant in his case. Once again, it was his process that was the primary focus of the sessions rather than the end product.

Alex

Though Alex could function at Piaget's pre-operational stage of development (2–7 Years), his sensory needs often kept him hovering mostly at the kinesthetic and sensory levels of the ETC. Intermittently, Alex would be able to move up to the perceptual and the cognitive levels where the image became a representation of something, but his great sensory needs seemed to minimise his emergence to the higher levels of the continuum. Although on occasion Alex was able to make associations with shapes and forms, name marks he made on paper and construct figures with play dough and plastic body parts, his engagement was not reflective of symbolic thought and remained at a concrete level. Hence, according to Lowenfeld's stages of artistic development Alex hovered between the scribble (2 years) and pre-schematic levels (4–6 years).

In one particular session, Alex seemed to function at the affective level of the ETC when he brought along a photograph of himself riding a horse and was very excited to show it off to me. Building on his excitement, I copied the photograph on the mirror and suggested we draw another one on paper. Alex eagerly held onto my hand as I assisted him to draw the horse with him sitting on top of the horse and proudly shared it with his mother after the session.

For Alex, the art product did hold some value, as in it facilitated longer cycles of engagement and functional communication between him and me and was a source of shared pleasure with his mother. However, it was secondary to his sensorial needs and was not the focus of the sessions.

Conclusion

The process of artmaking, call it pre-art or sensory play, is the focus of the S-BRATA, not necessarily the art product. That is not to say that the art product, if it were to emerge, does not hold value. It does in the case of the child who is at the developmental level of engaging, responding and reflecting upon it. However, with regards to children at the lower end of the spectrum who are not attentive to the marks they make and for whom the sensorial aspect of artmaking is primary, the product may not hold much value.

Tips

- Keep in mind the developmental stage of the child while artmaking.
- ETC may be used as a point of reference to gauge the level of art expression.
- Don't aim for an art product. It's okay if there is none.

References

Aach-Feldman, S., & Kunkle-Miller, C. (2016). Developmental art therapy. In Rubin, A. R. (Ed.), *Approaches to art therapy* (pp. 435–451). New York, NY: Routledge.

Charman, T. & Stone, W. (Eds.). (2006). *Social and communication development in autism spectrum disorders. early identification, diagnosis & intervention.* New York, NY: The Guilford Press.

Henley, R. (2018). *Creative response activities for children on the spectrum*. New York, NY: Routledge.

Lowenfeld, V. (1947). *Creative and mental growth*. New York, NY: Macmillan Co.

Lusebrink, V. B. (2016). Expressive therapies continuum. In Gussak, E. D. & Rosal, L. M. (Eds.), *The Wiley handbook of art therapy* (pp. 57–67). UK: Wiley- Blackwell.

Morgan, M. (Ed.). (1995). *Art 4-11. Art in the early years of Schooling*. Cheltenhem, UK: Stanley Thornes (Publishers) Ltd.

Piaget, J. (1954). *The construction of reality in the child*. New York, NY: Basic Books.

12 Conclusion

The research that led to the S-BRATA was instigated by my deep personal involvement with ASD by virtue of being the primary caregiver of a young adult with autism. Over a period of two decades, I sat through dozens of sessions of sensory integration therapy, speech and language therapy as well as other behavioral interventions with Moeez, integrating my learning with caregiving in addition to choosing a complementary career first as an educational therapist and later an art therapist.

As a novice art therapist, my very first clients were children with ASD and comorbid SID. I unconsciously tailored my intervention to address sensory issues in the children to lessen anxiety stemming from sensory challenges, to enable them to open up and engage with me through artmaking. The adverse impact of SID on sensory channels that mediate attachment behaviors between child and caregiver alerted me to the possibility of an impairment in the attachment patterns of children with autism, a high incidence of which is confirmed by research. The significance of a healthy attachment pattern and its vital impact on the child's psycho-emotional and developmental well-being instigated the notion of the therapist as an attachment figure who could concurrently address sensory regulation issues through the use of art materials. The urgency to highlight the importance of addressing the mental health of children on the spectrum was driven by the fact that their psycho-emotional well-being seems to take a back seat to ASD specific therapies that largely target the teaching of life skills and modifying behaviors. As a mother of an anxious teenager with ASD and having worked with equally anxious children as a therapist, I was faced with the nagging realisation that caregivers of the children were so overwhelmed by dealing with unwanted behaviors and developmental challenges that the mental health of the children did not receive the attention it deserved.

Research showed that old attachment patterns could be replaced with new ones later on in life, and that had implications for an intervention that could ameliorate the effects of a disrupted attachment (Siegel, 2003). In 2014, I published an article in the *Journal of Psychotherapy Integration* (Durrani, 2014) where I described a case study of a 12-year-old boy with ASD and significant SID. In that article, I illustrated how art therapy intervention had lowered anxiety levels in my client and facilitated attachment between him and me. I recommended further exploration of art therapy as a potential treatment for children with ASD. I also published a memoir by the name of *Wrapped in Blue* (2015), wherein I documented my journey of raising a child with autism with severe sensory challenges. In subsequent years, I felt there were gaps in my knowledge of theory and practice that could only be addressed through further research in art therapy within the context of ASD. Consequently, I pursued the doctorate in art therapy to bridge those gaps. The Sensory-Based Relational Art Therapy Approach (S-BRATA) is the fruit of the search for a deeper understanding of the work that I had been doing for many years.

S-BRATA is an empirical illustration of my learning from current research and practice in art therapy and ASD, as well as the advancement of that learning through the case studies of Teo, Raj and Alex. Each theme of the S-BRATA extends and develops some of the established concepts proposed by the art therapists who have worked with children with autism, some of whom I have referenced in this book. S-BRATA pushes the boundaries of art therapy practice, at times challenging the traditional approach by taking away the emphasis from the art product to focusing on the process. It also opens up the practice to the inclusion of elements from other arts-based disciplines.

Primary to the S-BRATA is the process of entering the child's inner world through engagement with art materials that are used to induce regulation and motivate the child to initiate communication with the therapist. The therapist is positioned as an attachment figure, and emulating an attachment relationship is fundamental to the objectives of the intervention. Hence, a session based on S-BRATA may not resemble a typical art therapy session where the interaction between therapist and child may be restricted to art-making on a single surface like a table or the floor or the creation of an art product. For instance, there may be entire sessions that are only dedicated to sensory play or activities other than artmaking just because the child is not ready or motivated to engage with art materials. Hence, flexibility in approach is emphasised and allows for inclusion of play, drama and music in the sessions when the therapist might need to attune to the child using different media. The aim of the therapist is to enter the world of the child on the child's terms.

The basic themes that underlie the S-BRATA are neither restrictive nor prescriptive but are meant to be used as a guide by art therapists. Each theme lends insight into the complexity of dealing with a wide spectrum of challenges that require an informed and attuned approach, for each child with ASD is unique and adjustment and adaptation of the content within the themes may be required. All seven themes run concurrent to each other and are not sequential in nature. For instance, the first theme, which is the sense of safety, must pervade all the sessions just as the therapist must at all times maintain flexibility in approach and aim for attachment formation through mirroring and attunement.

Some specific techniques illustrated in S-BRATA, such as the holding back and approach and retreat techniques, may be considered unique to the field of art therapy. Holding back refers to the withholding attitude of the therapist who refrains from any kind of direct engagement with the child and may sit in a corner of the room making art in the sight of the child but not initiating contact. This type of approach is recommended to instill a sense of safety in the child. Similarly, the approach, engage and retreat technique refers to alternate periods of engagement and disengagement with the child, preventing sensory overload. For instance, the therapist needs to step back and give the child downtime to recoup and regulate if a certain activity has continued for long and may have overwhelmed the child. The above-mentioned techniques emanate from the implicit processes of embodied intelligence and interpersonal connectedness that facilitate a sense of awareness in the therapist of the emotional state of the child (Belkofer & Nolan, 2016; Kossak, 2009).

Self-Care and Supervision

The topics of self-care and supervision are much too vast for me to do any justice to them in this book; however, I feel it is important to at least bring some attention to them as both play a pivotal role in maintaining quality of practice and standard of care in the mental health profession. Self-care and supervision go hand in hand as both are not mutually exclusive and the therapist's own mental health has an impact on the work that she does and vice versa.

Whether one is a novice therapist or an experienced one, supervision provides a sounding board in the form of the supervisor with whom clinical, ethical and administrative questions and challenges can be addressed. In fact, supervisors are the "gatekeepers and guides" (Fish, 2017, p. 6) that oversee quality of care to the clients and help therapists keep things on track and avoid blind spots. They can also play the role of mentors, providing necessary insight and guidance as well validating the important work that therapists do.

During my work with Teo, Raj and Alex, I sought regular supervision to gain insight and clarity into multiple aspects of my intervention. There were issues of countertransference that needed to be addressed, periods of frustration at not being able to have a breakthrough, instances where I felt a lack of confidence or belief in the approach I was taking and so many other aspects of my practice that I needed to sound out and process with an expert who was able to look at my work objectively and from a distance. At times, therapists can get so entangled within the complex layers of interpersonal work that another set of eyes may be necessary to unravel and bring clarity to the different facets of clinical work. Often a fresh perspective can be illuminating and provide much needed direction and support.

In my sessions with Teo, there were many occasions where I felt stuck, frustrated and hopeless. When Teo did not acknowledge my presence for almost half of the 12 sessions I had with him, I began to question my belief in my intervention. My countertransference toward him was that of a mother desperately wanting response from her child, but I did not have the luxury of time with Teo as I had had with my own son. Hence, I had to manage my expectations and slow down. I discussed my reservations with my supervisor who has extensive experience working with individuals on the spectrum. She validated my feelings and encouraged me to persevere with patience and a realistic outlook. Her support reinforced my belief and self-confidence, and I was able to keep going with optimism.

The fact is that even the most experienced of therapists requires supervision and consultation or maybe even personal therapy to deal with confusion, anxiety, discomfort and vicarious trauma when facing personal or client problems (Ethical Principles for Art Therapists, 2013). Not addressing these issues may amount to self-harm and substandard professional services.

Personal therapy may not be necessary but is a form of self-care that should be taken seriously if the need presents itself. Burnout is not uncommon among therapists when working with high stress clients or working long hours. Therapists simply cannot afford to be neglectful of their own psycho-emotional health as they are the containers and holders of their client's emotional baggage, and if they themselves are not emotionally grounded, they could likely compromise their professional and ethical standards. Whereas clinical supervision is mainly for case related or administrative work, personal therapy is where the roles are reversed and the therapist allows him- or herself to be held and supported emotionally.

Response Art

Along with personal therapy and supervision, art therapists have the privilege of using response art to express, process and gain insight into clinical and personal matters. Response art does not have to be the domain of art therapists only, and other professionals can benefit from it as well through art-based supervision. Fish (2017) asserted that response art is a means to "reflect and communicate the therapist's understanding of the client's experience, provide client feedback in session, and empathize with the client's experience during or after session" (p. 31). Response art does not only facilitate a deeper understanding of the client, it can also be employed as a form of self-care for the therapist. Allen (2014) in her book *Art Is a Way of Knowing: A Guide to Self-Knowledge and Spiritual Fulfillment Through Creativity* expounds the potential of artmaking to connect with the deepest aspects of our selves that require attention. Thus, response art can become the conduit for any kind of expression the therapist may be seeking for clarity, direction or insight, whether for professional or personal reasons.

The data that generated the S-BRATA do not include the response art I made during the duration of the research as it was beyond my scope to handle such a large body of information in addition to all the videos and clinical notes.

However, I made art intermittently to process some difficult sessions with Alex, Raj and Teo that helped me externalise the confusion and frustration I felt at times and also to get a sense of what the boys may be experiencing in the sessions. For example, Figure 12.1 was my attempt to understand Teo's enclosed world where the small hand represents him wanting to reach out and connect despite his challenges. The larger hand behind Teo's is my hand, offering him validation and support by mirroring him and holding him amidst the cacophony of sensory overload.

Figure 12.2 was made in response to Raj, in which I was trying to capture the constant movement that pervaded my sessions with him. The red square represents the art therapy studio and the blue lines depict Raj running back and forth along the edges of the room. The handprints going in different directions are my attempt to contain Raj. The entire image is reflective of my sense of being all over the place and not being able to contain Raj's anxiety.

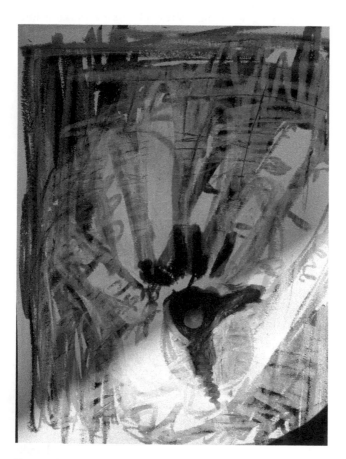

Figure 12.1 Response art Teo

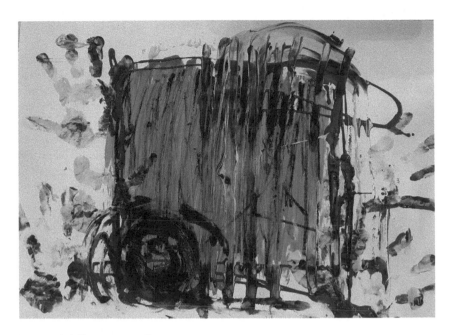

Figure 12.2 Response art Raj

Recommendations for Further Development of the Framework

Although my research focuses specifically on working with children on the spectrum who have sensory issues and impaired attachment, the framework is not exclusive to this population. It has the potential of wider applicability, and practitioners are encouraged to adapt and develop it to suit their client's needs. Again, S-BRATA does not have to be the exclusive domain of art therapists. Expressive therapies practitioners such as dance, music, movement and drama therapists, professionals who incorporate sensory, kinesthetic, tactile, visual and auditory elements in their work, can also employ the basic principles of S-BRATA in their approaches. In fact, a collaboration between art therapists and other expressive therapies practitioners could enhance the framework with cross-disciplinary learning and sharing.

In a recent study conducted on the mental health and parental practices of caregivers of children with ASD, Teague, Newman, Tonge, and Gray (2018) contend that the caregivers require support to improve their caregiving skills, which have implications for quality of attachment between them and the child. They add, "[C]aregivers may benefit from interventions that assist them to identify and interpret their child's subjective state, and effectively communicate with their children with ASD" (p. 2650).

Subsequent to the termination of my sessions with Teo, Raj and Alex, I worked with a 14-year-old boy Ali (pseudonym) who was on the spectrum. Ali was nonverbal and his receptive language was limited to single commands, to which he responded inconsistently. Ali was a heavily built teenager who was unaware of his strength and would sometimes use it on others. He would punch his head when frustrated, and these episodes could occur without any perceivable triggers. Ali's mother Ayesha requested to sit in the sessions accompanied by the helper Umi, who assisted her with Ali's caregiving. I agreed to let both Ayesha and Umi sit in the therapy room, initially just for observation. Post-session discussions with Ayesha revealed her disconnect with Ali and her discomfort in interacting with him. Gauging the lack of insight Ayesha had in engaging with her child, I explained the theoretical basis of my interaction with Ali as I modeled the S-BRATA for her so that she could understand what I was doing with him and why. I would begin the session by playing catch with Ali, then move on to sensory art making with his favorite art material: paint. I alternated between paint and crayons to manage Ali's arousal levels. Often Ali would break the crayons into two or peel their stickers and I allowed him to do that, sensing his need for deep proprioceptive input. When Ayesha got perturbed by Ali's actions and, according to her, making more mess than "real art," I addressed her concerns in light of his developmental level and sensory needs. As the sessions progressed, I invited Ayesha and Umi to participate in the sessions and do joint artmaking as well as by including them in the play between myself and Ali. When I asked Ayesha for feedback on Ali's progress and whether she had gained anything from being a part of the sessions, she shared she had benefitted a lot from observing me work with him and gained a deeper understanding of her son.

One could argue that S-BRATA encompasses less than or more than the scope of art therapy and is not in fact art therapy due to its broad and flexible elements. In my opinion, strict categorisation limits the scope of the intervention and is unnecessary. It is hoped that further research by art therapists will contribute to the evidence base of S-BRATA through ongoing quantitative and qualitative research as it has significant implications for inclusion in the treatment of children on the autism spectrum, especially within the context of psychological and emotional well-being. Due to the limitations of my study, I was unable to include caregivers in my sessions with my subjects. Dyadic sessions facilitated by the art therapist, such as I conducted with Ali and Ayesha, hold exciting possibilities for research and development within the context of attachment between caregiver and child with ASD.

References

Allen, B. P. (2014). *Art is a way of knowing*. Boston, MA: Shambala.

Belkofer, C. M., & Nolan, E. (2016). Practical applications of neuroscience in art therapy: A holistic approach to treating Trauma in Children. In King, L. J. (Ed). *Art therapy, trauma, and neuroscience* (pp. 157–172). New York, NY: Routledge.

Durrani, H. (2014). Facilitating attachment in children with autism through art therapy: A case study. *Journal of Psychotherapy Integration*, 24(2), 99. 10.1037/a0036974.

Durrani, H. (2015). *Wrapped in blue*. Partridge India.

Ethical Principles for Art Therapists (2013). Retrieved from: https://arttherapy.org/wp-content/uploads/2017/06/Ethical-Principles-for-Art-Therapists.pdfs.

Fish, J. B. (2017). *Art-based supervision. Cultivating therapeutic insight through imagery*. New York, NY: Routledge.

Kossak, M. S. (2009). Therapeutic attunement: A transpersonal view of expressive arts therapy. *The Arts in Psychotherapy*, 36, 13–18. doi: 10.1016/j.aip.2008.09.003.

Teague, J. S., Newman, K. L., Tonge, J. B., & Gray, K. M. (2018). Caregiver mental health, parenting practices, and perceptions of child attachment in children with autism spectrum disorder. *Journal of Autism and Developmental Disorders*, 48, 2642–2652. https://doi.org/10.1007/s10803-018-3517-x.

Index

9 780367 442262